D0918987

Nutrition and Aerobic Exercise

ACS SYMPOSIUM SERIES **294**

Nutrition and Aerobic Exercise

Donald K. Layman, EDITOR
University of Illinois at Urbana–Champaign

American Chemical Society, Washington, D.C. 1986

Library of Congress Cataloging in Publication Data

Nutrition and aerobic exercise.
(ACS symposium series, ISSN 0097–6156; 294)

Developed from a symposium held Apr. 10, 1984, in
St. Louis, entitled "The Influence of Aerobic Exercise
on Energy Metabolism and Nutrient Requirements",
sponsored by the Division of Agricultural and Food
Chemistry of the American Chemical Society, the
Quaker Oats Company, and the Dart-Kraft Company.

Includes bibliographies and index.

Contents: Nutrition and exercise/ Donald K.
Layman—Biochemical adaptations in skeletal muscle
induced by exercise training/ Ronald L. Terjung and
David A. Hood—Influence of aerobic exercise on fuel
utilization/ Michael N. Goodman—[etc.]

1. Nutrition—Congresses. 2. Exercise—Physiological
aspects—Congresses.

I. Layman, Donald K., 1950-   . II. American
Chemical Society. Division of Agricultural and Food
Chemistry. III. Quaker Oats Company. IV. Dart &
Kraft. V. Series.

QP141.A1N86155   1986   612'.3   85–26872
ISBN 0–8412–0949–9

ACS Symposium Series

M. Joan Comstock, *Series Editor*

Advisory Board

FOREWORD

The ACS SYMPOSIUM SERIES was founded in 1974 to provide a medium for publishing symposia quickly in book form. The format of the Series parallels that of the continuing ADVANCES IN CHEMISTRY SERIES except that, in order to save time, the papers are not typeset but are reproduced as they are submitted by the authors in camera-ready form. Papers are reviewed under the supervision of the Editors with the assistance of the Series Advisory Board and are selected to maintain the integrity of the symposia; however, verbatim reproductions of previously published papers are not accepted. Both reviews and reports of research are acceptable, because symposia may embrace both types of presentation.

CONTENTS

PREFACE

THE POTENTIAL HEALTH BENEFITS of a combined program of nutrition and exercise have increasingly been recognized during the past decade. World-class athletes have long known the importance of controlling caloric intake to maintain desired body weight and that a poor diet will diminish performance. However, as the general public becomes more conscious of health and fitness, routine aerobic exercise is becoming a focal point of daily health maintenance for large numbers of people. This trend raises new questions about the impact of exercise on nutritional requirements. This book addresses the principal questions concerning the interaction of nutrition and aerobic exercise training. Each chapter reviews the basic topics and examines new findings and important questions remaining to be solved.

The book is written for an audience that has a basic understanding of physiology and intermediary metabolism. However, it assumes little or no background in nutrition or exercise physiology. It is intended to provide an easily read insight into the current knowledge about nutrition and exercise, and it should appeal to both the specialist and nonspecialist.

This book originated from a symposium entitled "The Influence of Aerobic Exercise on Energy Metabolism and Nutrient Requirements" and was sponsored by the Division of Agricultural and Food Chemistry of the American Chemical Society, the Quaker Oats Company, and the Dart-Kraft Company. I would like to especially thank John Whitaker, David Hurt, and Robert Bursey as the representatives of the respective sponsors.

DONALD K. LAYMAN
University of Illinois
Urbana, IL 61801

September 19, 1985

Nutrition and Exercise: An Overview

Donald K. Layman

Department of Foods and Nutrition, Division of Nutritional Sciences, University of Illinois, Urbana, IL 61801

Across the United States, interest has increased in physical fitness, exercise, and nutrition. Almost one-half of adult Americans state that they exercise regularly (1). Activities include walking, running, swimming, biking, racketball, tennis, aerobic dancing, and many others. The renewed interest in exercise appears to be due, in large part, to the association of exercise with health. Most health organizations, including the American Heart Association, the American Diabetes Association, the American Dietetic Association, and the American Medical Association, advocate exercise for maintenance of health and to reduce the risk of the onset of the adult diseases of obesity, hypertension, heart disease, and diabetes (2-4).

Likewise, health-related changes have occurred in the American diet. The Dietary Goals for the United States developed in 1977 by the Senate Select Committee on Nutrition (5) recommended that adults reduce their calorie intake, reduce total fat, saturated fat, and cholesterol, avoid excessive salt intake, and increase consumption of complex carbohydrates and fiber. These recommendations have resulted in trends toward lower consumption of animal products plus use of low fat products and increased consumption of fruits and vegetables. Consumers are selecting less sugar and saturated fat (6). During the past 3 years, use of poultry and fish has increased about 16%, while use of beef and eggs has decreased 16% (7). This increased consciousness of the general public to nutrition has also led to a proliferation of miracle diets, quick weight loss schemes, and vitamin supplements. Surveys indicate that the majority of Americans take vitamin supplements (6) and many have tried a fad weight loss diet (8).

The response of the American public to utilize diet and exercise for maintenance of health has increased the need for more definitive scientific information about the interactions of exercise with dietary needs. This book reviews some of the physiological and metabolic changes that occur during exercise training and examines the impact of routine exercise on nutritional requirements.

Physiological and Metabolic Responses to Exercise

The influence of physical activity on nutritional requirements and
health is not the same for all activities. For the purposes of this
book, exercise will be classified as either anaerobic or aerobic
activities. These terms provide descriptive information about both
the level of exertion and the duration of the activity and are
useful in relating activities to nutritional needs. Anaerobic
exercise includes activities such as weightlifting and sprinting,
and involves maximum exertion for periods of time less than 1 or 2
minutes. Aerobic activities are performed for periods usually in
excess of 15 minutes at less than maximum speed or strength.
Aerobic exercise requires greater endurance and includes activities
such as distance running, swimming, biking, and walking.
      Some of the responses by the body to anaerobic exercise are
visually obvious. Greater strength, speed, and muscle development
are reasons that athletes emphasize anaerobic training. However,
research has shown that these results are not easily predicted, and
even the effects on the amount of muscle mass are not entirely clear
(9). The effects of these short-duration exercises on
cardiopulmonary function and on nutritional requirements are minimal.
      Aerobic exercise involves endurance training. As the body
performs activities for extended periods, physiological and cellular
adaptations occur (10-12). These adaptations focus on the ability
of the body to supply oxygen to the muscle cells, the capacity of
the cells to utilize oxygen, and a shift in the fuel source to
greater use of fatty acids. The magnitude of these changes defines
aerobic capacity and endurance.
      Aerobic training produces numerous physiological changes,
including changes in heart rate and oxygen uptake. There is a
decrease in the resting heart rate and the heart rate at any
specific work load. However, cardiac output is maintained because
stroke volume is increased. Changes also occur within the muscle
cells that allow for increased oxygen uptake from the circulating
blood. Thus, aerobic exercise training increases stroke volume, the
efficiency of oxygen uptake by muscles (A-V O_2), VO_2 max and reduces
the heart rate during submaximal exercise (10,13-14).
      At the cellular level, aerobic exercise training increases the
oxidative capacity of the tissues (11), and produces numerous
changes in the function of the muscle cells. Changes in specific
skeletal muscle cells and the effects of exercise intensity,
duration, and frequency are discussed in Chapter 2. Mitochondria
increase in size and number which allows for increased oxygen use in
fuel conversion to energy for muscular contraction. Training also
produces a shift in the primary source of fuel for exercise from
carbohydrates to fatty acids. Since fatty acids are the principal
form of fuel storage in the body, this shift is critical in allowing
for prolonged activity. Use of carbohydrates and lipids during
aerobic exercise is examined in Chapter 3.

Influence of Aerobic Exercise on Nutritional Needs

Interest in the relationship of nutrition and exercise arises from
many sources. Athletes and coaches often seek an extra edge from
specific foods or supplements. Wrestlers, dancers, and gymnasts

frequently attempt to control food intake to modify body weight;
and, as stated above, large numbers of people are now looking to the
combination of improved nutrition and exercise for maintenance of
health. Thus, the topics of "Nutrition and Exercise" produce a wide
variety of questions from a diverse audience with different needs
and goals. Questions most frequently asked include:

> Is exercise important for weight control?
> Is increased protein essential for muscle building or
>   strength?
> Does exercise reduce the risk of heart disease?
> Should athletes take vitamin supplements?
> Are salt tablets or electrolyte drinks essential for
>   exercise during hot weather?
> Is exercise important for a diabetic?
> Does aerobic exercise create an increased need for iron?
> Does exercise prevent osteoporosis?

This book addresses these issues and examines the current research
in these areas.

To evaluate nutrition requirements, the reader needs a basic
understanding of nutrients and the parameters that affect their
needs. Nutrients are chemical substances needed to maintain life
which are supplied to the body in food or drinks. The nutrients
include vitamins, minerals, carbohydrates, fats, proteins, and
water. These classifications of nutrients encompass approximately
45 different chemicals that are involved in every function or
structure of the body. While some of these functions that are
directly influenced by exercise will be discussed in the subsequent
chapters, a complete listing of these functions is beyond the scope
of this book. For a more thorough review of nutrient functions, the
reader is referred to any one of a number of excellent nutrition
references (5-6,15-16).

To assess the impact of exercise on the needs for specific
nutrients, nutrient functions must be evaluated. At a generalized
level, the functions of nutrients are (a) growth or maintenance of
the structures of the body (one can consider either macro-structures
like muscles and bones, or micro-structures like cell membranes and
enzymes), (b) fuels for the energy to run the body processes, (c)
fluids and regulation of body fluids, and (d) protection from toxic
substances including toxic chemicals, carcinogens, and antigens.
The effects of exercise on nutritional requirements can be assessed
against the likelihood of substantial changes in one or more of
these functions.

As the effects of exercise on the body are examined, clearly
the primary effects are on body fluids and fuels. Movement of the
body requires additional fuels and the process of conversion of
these fuels into energy produces heat which must be dissipated, in
large part, by evaporation of sweat from the skin.

Water is the most critical of the effects of exercise on
nutritional requirements. As discussed in Chapter 8, exercise
produces increased body heat and increased water losses. If this
results in dehydration, it will decrease performance and can produce
nausea, irregularities in heart beat, heat stroke, and death.
Associated with water losses, there are losses of salts or

electrolytes. However, water loss is clearly the most limiting
factor for work capacity as defined in a position paper by the
American College of Sports Medicine (17).

After supplying an adequate amount of water, the next most
important dietary issue is adequate energy. Physical activity is
the major variable of energy expenditure and the only component
under voluntary control. The other components are basal metabolism
(the energy expended to maintain the vital body processes while at
rest) and Specific Dynamic Action (the energy utilized during the
digestion, absorption, and assimilation of nutrients after a meal).
These two components expend about 1000-2000 kilocalories of energy
per day, depending on the size of the body and composition of
meals. However, food intakes range from 2000 to 6000 kcals per day,
depending on the level of activity. Sedentary adults need about
2000-2500 kcal/day, while athletes consume approximately 3000-4000
kcal/day (18). The primary factors determining the energy
expenditure of exercise are the weight of the body and the distance
traveled. While it is true that there is less energy expended at
walking speeds versus running due to greater efficiencies in
movement, over a fairly wide range of running speeds energy
expenditure is essentially independent of speed for a given distance
(19-20).

Fuels for the body are limited to carbohydrates, fats, and
proteins. In the American diet, these fuels are consumed in a ratio
of approximately 46:42:12 with the recommended ratio being closer to
53:35:12 (5). Thus in a nongrowing adult, these ratios provide
estimates of the fuel use for daily activities. The primary fuels
for exercise are carbohydrates and fats. Chapter 3 examines
utilization of specific fuels during aerobic exercise. As the
amount of daily exercise increases, there is an increased energy
expenditure and hence increased need for energy nutrients usually
reflected in increased food consumption, decreased body fat, or both
(see Chapter 9).

Protein has long been a dominant feature at the training table
for athletes who believe that high intakes of protein are essential
for muscle development and strength. However, research indicates
that little or no additional protein is required for maximum muscle
growth. Interestingly, recent studies suggest that aerobic exercise
may have larger effects on protein metabolism than anaerobic
training (21). The effects of both anaerobic and aerobic exercise
on the nutritional needs for protein are reviewed in Chapter 4.

As discussed above, aerobic exercise produces numerous
physiologic and metabolic changes in the body. Many of these
changes are believed to be beneficial for prevention of heart
disease. The effects on cardiopulmonary function were mentioned
earlier and are clearly beneficial, as are the changes in body
composition described in Chapter 9. Further, aerobic exercise
appears to have positive effects on blood cholesterol and other
lipids. These effects of exercise on the metabolism of lipids and
the important transport particles called lipoproteins are discussed
in Chapter 5.

Athletes have long sought to maximize performance by use of
special nutrients. "Ergogenic Aids" have been promoted to increase
endurance, strength, or performance. Ergogenic aids including
vitamins, minerals, and other substances are suggested to "supply"

or "produce" more energy. Besides pure vitamin and mineral supplements, other aids include honey, wheat germ oil, gelatin, glucose, and vitamin E. With the exception of possible psychological benefits, any other suggested benefits are without sound scientific documentation (22). As with most misleading advertising, the premise begins with a basic fact and then plays to the desires of the consumer. For example, conventional wisdom holds that the requirements of many of the B-vitamins are dependent on the amount of energy or number of calories used by the body. For thiamin, riboflavin, niacin, pantothenic acid, and biotin, the needs could increase proportional to energy expenditure. Thus the athlete burning twice the energy of the non-athlete was assumed to have approximately twice the B-vitamin needs. While the "logic" that exercise increases B-vitamin needs is reasonable, only riboflavin has been specifically studied. Chapter 6 summarizes these findings and indicates that while riboflavin needs are increased, the increase is small and the associated increased food consumption should be adequate to meet these needs without supplementation.

The effects of exercise on the dietary needs for minerals have not been extensively studied. Of particular interest is the impact of exercise on the minerals iron and calcium which are examined in Chapter 7. Iron is an essential component of hemoglobin which is responsible for transport of oxygen within red blood cells in the blood. Thus, iron deficiency (anemia) will decrease oxygen carrying capacity of the blood and hence lower aerobic capacity. This problem appears to be most important for women who frequently have marginal iron intakes (5).

Calcium needs and metabolism have become an important nutrition issue due to the increased prevalence of osteoporosis. Osteoporosis is a disease of fragility of major bones such as the pelvis, femur, and spine caused by an age-related loss of bone minerals. As discussed in Chapter 7, calcium intake and physical activity may favorably affect the calcium content of bones and delay the onset of osteoporosis.

These issues and associated topics are discussed in more detail in the following chapters. Each of the individual authors has provided background information and research data in an effort to review and evaluate the important issues. Finally, each author has provided a summary statement defining the nutrient needs during an aerobic exercise program.

Literature Cited

1. U.S. Department of Health, Education, and Welfare. (1979) Healthy people. The Surgeon General's report on health promotion and disease prevention. DHEW (PHS) Publ. No. 79-55071.

2. American Heart Association. (December, 1981) Statement on Exercise. Springfield, IL.

3. American Dietetic Association. (1980) Nutrition and physical fitness. J. Am. Diet. Assoc. 76, 437.

4. Castelli, W. P. (1979) Exercise and high-density lipoproteins (editorial). J. Am. Med. Assoc. 242, 2217.

5. Guthrie, H. A. (1983) Introductory Nutrition. 5th edition. C. V. Mosby Co., St. Louis.

6. Hamilton, E. M., Whitney, E. N. & Sizer, F. S. (1985) In: Nutrition: Concepts and Controversies. West Publishing Co., St. Paul.

7. American Institute for Cancer Research. (Summer, 1985) Trends in Food Consumption. In: AICR Newsletter. Falls Church, VA.

8. Stern, J. S. (1983) Diet and Exercise. In: Obesity (Greenwood, M.R.C., ed.), pp. 65-84, Churchill Livingstone, New York.

9. Clark, D. H. (1973) Adaptations in strength and muscular endurance resulting from exercise. Exer. Sport Sci. Rev. 1, 73-102.

10. McArdle, W. D., Katch, F. I. & Katch, V. L. (1981) Exercise Physiology: Energy, Nutrition, and Performance. Lea & Febiger, Philadelphia.

11. Holloszy, J. O. & Booth, F. W. (1976) Biochemical adaptations to endurance exercise in muscle. Ann. Rev. Physiol. 38, 273-291.

12. Pollock, M. L. (1973) The quantification of endurance training programs. Exer. Sport Sci. Rev. 1, 155-188.

13. Saltin, B. (1973) Metabolic fundamentals in exercise. Med. Sci. Sports 5, 137-146.

14. Keul, J. (1973) The relationship between circulation and metabolism during exercise. Med. Sci. Sports 5, 209-219.

15. Briggs, G. M. & Calloway, D. H. (1979) Nutrition and Physical Fitness. 10th edition. W. B. Saunders Co., Philadelphia.

16. Pike, R. L. & Brown, M. L. (1984) Nutrition: An integrated approach. 3rd edition. John Wiley & Sons, New York.

17. American College of Sports Medicine. (1975) Position Paper. Med. Sci. Sports 7:7.

18. Buskirk, E. R. (1981) Some nutritional considerations in the conditioning of athletes. Ann. Rev. Nutr. 1, 319-350.

19. Fellingham, G. W., Roundy, E. S., Fisher, A. G. & Bryce, G. R. (1978) Caloric cost of walking and running. Med. Sci. Sports 10, 132-136.

20. Howley, E. T. & Glover, M. E. (1974) The caloric cost of running and walking one mile for men and women. Med. Sci. Sports 6, 235-237.

21. Lemon, P.W.R. & Nagle, F. J. (1981) Effects of exercise on protein and amino acid metabolism. Med. Sci. Sports 13, 141-149.

22. Williams, M. H. (1985) Ergogenic foods. In: Nutritional Aspects of Human Physical and Athletic Performance. 2nd edition, pp. 296-321, Charles C. Thomas, Springfield, IL.

RECEIVED September 6, 1985

2

Biochemical Adaptations in Skeletal Muscle Induced by Exercise Training

Ronald L. Terjung and David A. Hood

Department of Physiology, Upstate Medical Center, State University of New York, Syracuse, NY 13210

Exercise performance seems to be greatly affected by the chronic level of physical activity experienced by the animal or individual. For example, differences in the capacity for prolonged exercise seem obvious between wild and domesticated animals. This is probably due, in part, to inherent biochemical differences between the muscles of active and less active species (1). Muscles of wild animals appear darker than those of their domesticated counterparts (2). Further, variations in activity patterns due to seasonal change (3) or hibernation (4), are associated with differences in the enzymes related to oxidative metabolism. Thus, in a general sense physical activity seems to be associated with biochemical changes that enhance the muscle's capacity for aerobic metabolism.

Muscle Adaptations

The specific biochemical changes induced by increased physical activity are well characterized from laboratory studies and have been the subject of a number of excellent reviews (5-9). The fundamental change found in skeletal muscle after exercise training is an enhanced capacity for energy provision via aerobic metabolism. There is an increase in mitochondrial protein content and cristae component enzymes associated with the electron transport. In a thorough study, Holloszy (10) found that an exercise program of prolonged treadmill running increased the mitochondrial content of laboratory rats by approximately 100%. Similar training responses are found in a wide variety of other animals including man (9,11). Subsequent morphological studies have shown that the mitochondria of trained muscles appear to be more abundant (12) and larger (13). Thus, the cross-section of the trained muscle appears more densely packed with mitochondria. Mitochondria isolated from muscles of trained animals exhibit the same dependence on ADP to stimulate and increase respiration, and are as efficient in the coupling of ATP production to oxygen consumption as muscle obtained from sedentary animals (10). Thus, the increased mitochondrial content represents a true increase in the potential for aerobic ATP generation within the muscle. In addition to the greater electron transport capacity, there is also a coordinated increase in the enzymes of support

0097-6156/86/0294-0008$06.00/0

systems necessary to supply the reducing equivalents for the electron transport and ATP synthesis. Thus, the capacities for carbohydrate oxidation (14), fatty acid oxidation (15,16), ketone body
oxidation (17), tricarboxylic acid cycle enzymes (18), and mitochondrial shuttle pathways (19) are increased by endurance training.
In addition, the content of myoglobin, which is thought to facilitate oxygen transfer within the cell (20,21), increases in the
trained muscle (2,22). Thus, there is a coordinated increase in the
capacity of the trained muscle for ATP provision via oxidative
metabolism. These changes contribute to the darker appearing
muscles of the trained animals. The primary metabolic significance
of the enhanced aerobic capacity is probably related to the control
of energy metabolism and a shift in substrate source from carbohydrate to fat in the muscles during submaximal exercise (6,8,23).

Specificity of Adaptations

The biochemical adaptations to exercise training are very specific
to the working muscles. For example, an increase is found in the
hindlimb muscle of treadmill run rats, but not in liver (24) or the
less active abdominal muscles of the same animals (22). Further,
when a unique training program that exercises only one limb on a
cycle ergometer is employed, the adaptation is induced in the
exercised leg, but not the untrained contralateral leg (13,25).
Thus, the training adaptation is not a generalized response within
the individual. This indicates that the stimulus responsible for
bringing about the biochemical change is specific to the working
muscle and related to the demands placed upon the muscle by the
exercise effort.
    Factors that determine the magnitude of the training effect are
fairly complex, due in part to the ordered pattern of motor unit
recruitment found during normal locomotion and/or a specific work
task. The type and intensity of the exercise effort largely determine which motor units will be utilized to perform the work (26).
Each motor unit within a muscle is composed of a single nerve axon
and the muscle fibers that it innervates. While all fibers within a
given motor unit have the same properties, it is now recognized that
at least three different skeletal muscle fiber types (and thus motor
units) exist in mammals. They differ considerably in their contractile characteristics, in their inherent biochemical capabilities,
and probably in their response to training. Thus, it is important
to consider the impact of the different types of skeletal muscle
motor units.

Muscle Fiber Types

Mammalian skeletal muscle can be separated into two distinct fiber
populations, based on relative contraction characteristics, and are
referred to as slow-twitch (Type I) or fast-twitch (Type II) fibers.
The slow-twitch fiber type exhibits a relatively low shortening
velocity (27), a low rate of tension development (27), a low myosin
ATPase activity (28) and a low rate of calcium sequestration by the
sarcoplasmic reticulum (29). The converse is true for the fast-
twitch fibers. Since contraction velocity highly correlates with
myosin ATPase activity (30), it is possible to easily identify,

within a muscle cross-section, fast and slow-twitch fibers by the intensity of staining of the myosin ATPase using histochemical procedures (31). The slow-twitch fibers are characteristically red in appearance, indicative of a relatively high mitochondrial content (14), exhibit a high blood flow (32,33), and have a low glycogenolytic capacity (e.g., phosphorylase activity) (7,34). The fast-twitch fibers uniformly possess a relatively high glycogenolytic capacity (7,34), but can be subdivided by their contrasting capacities for oxidative metabolism. In fact, the greatest difference in mitochondrial content for most non-primate mammalian muscle is found between the fast-twitch red and the fast-twitch white fiber types (14,35). In humans, the mitochondrial content of slow-twitch red fibers is typically greater than that of the fast-twitch red fibers (7,35). Similarly, measurements of blood flows to sections of muscle, which are primarily composed of a single fiber type, exhibit large differences consistent with the expected demands of oxygen supply based on mitochondrial content (32,33). Thus, mammalian skeletal muscle is typically comprised of three biochemically and functionally distinct fiber types: slow-twitch red, fast-twitch red and fast-twitch white. These fiber types are also commonly referred to as Type I, Type IIa, and Type IIb, respectively (7).

Contraction performance of these different fiber types is predictable from a knowledge of their biochemical and blood flow differences. For example, the slow-twitch red fiber type can contract for long periods of time without a loss in tension development (36). Although the relatively high functional aerobic capacity must be important for sustained performance (37), it is also known that the slow-twitch fiber type requires less energy to maintain tension (38). Therefore, this fiber type seems well-suited for prolonged sustained activity such as that required for postural support. The fast-twitch red muscle fiber is fairly fatigue resistant and capable of repeated powerful contractions before tension development declines significantly (36). Although this fiber type has a high capacity for lactate production (39,40), its performance during prolonged contraction periods is made possible by its relatively high functional aerobic capacity (40). In contrast, the fast-twitch white muscle fiber exhibits a rapid loss of tension development and is capable of powerful contractions for only a brief period of time (36). A high rate of glycogenolysis, resulting in a high lactate content and cellular acidosis, would be found during intense contraction conditions in this fiber type (41).

The slow-twitch muscle fibers are relatively small in diameter and belong to motor units that are typically the first to be recruited during any motor task. Thus, during simple muscle activity required for postural support of standing, the slow-twitch motor units are very active and, in some cases, function near their maximal force output (42). The fast-twitch red fibers belong to larger motor units (26) and are recruited for muscle actions that are more forceful (42). Their recruitment increases, for example, when running at increasing speeds on a treadmill (42). Finally, the fast-twitch white fibers belong to large powerful motor units and are recruited during very intense exercise (43,44) or during extremely forceful movements such as jumping (42). The relatively infrequent and specialized utilization of the fast-twitch white motor units is especially purposeful, since these intense exercise efforts and explosive body movements are usually short lived. Thus, the rapid fatigue and relatively poor endurance performance of this fiber type (36) do not generally influence muscle function during moderate exercise of submaximal intensity (43,44). Athough there can be a significant overlap in the progressive recruitment of motor unit populations as the intensity of exercise becomes greater, the general pattern of ordered recruitment from slow-twitch red to fast-twitch red and then to fast-twitch white motor units occurs during most physical activity (45). The skeletal musculature of those non-primate mammals that have been examined is comprised primarily of (i.e., 80-95%) fast-twitch fibers (46,47). The fast-twitch fibers are, in turn, comprised of approximately equal portions of fast-twitch red and fast-twitch white fibers. In contrast the skeletal muscle of man is comprised of approximately 50% fast-twitch and 50% slow-twitch muscle (7,48). Although the low-oxidative fast-twitch white muscle fibers are found in humans (7,49), they typically represent a smaller fraction of the limb musculature as compared to most lower mammals.

In summary, all mammals possess a large fraction of high-oxidative muscle. The ordered pattern of motor unit recruitment involves these high oxidative muscle fibers before the low-oxidative fibers, as exercise intensity progresses from mild, to moderate, to severe. This progression favors an enhanced exercise performance at submaximal exercise intensities, since the slow and fast-twitch red fibers are capable of repeated contractions for long periods of time.

Important Training Parameters

Several important training variables are known to influence the magnitude of the biochemical response. These include the duration of the training program, the intensity of the exercise effort, the duration of each exercise bout (minutes/day), and the frequency of exercise (i.e., days/week).

Training Duration. It is intuitively obvious that the duration of training must be sufficiently long for the maximal response to be developed. This is due, in part, to the nature of most training programs that typically progress from relatively mild or moderate exercise efforts to the more intense exercise bouts that will be maintained thereafter. Thus, the cellular stimulus for adaptation is probably continually changing until the peak exercise effort, that will be routinely sustained for the steady state training program, is achieved. After this time the full training response might be expected. However, there is an additional time delay before realizing the full adaptive change. This additional time is due to the cellular events associated with the adaptive response within the cell. In the case of a biochemical change of an increase in mitochondrial protein, the fully developed response, representing the steady state change within the muscle fiber, is dependent upon the cellular dynamics of protein turnover. Specifically, the rate at which a new steady state concentration of mitochondria occurs within the muscle is dependent upon the degradation rate constant of the mitochondrial components (50). Since protein degradation is a first-order process, the time course of mitochondrial content change is non-linear and is conveniently considered in terms of half-life. In this context, the half-life can be considered as the time required for the mitochondrial content to proceed through one-half the change, from the existing value, toward the new steady state value determined by the training stimulus. Although it is probable that the turnover of mitochondria does not occur at the same rate in all muscle fiber types (51), an average half-life of approximately 1 week is a reasonable value for mixed muscle of animals (52,53) and man (54). Thus, even if the cellular stimulus, sufficient to increase cytochrome c to double that normally found, were to occur instantaneously and remain constant thereafter, only one-half of the response would be measured when training proceeded for the next week. Training the subsequent week would then produce another one-half of the effect, to bring the response to 75% completion. Each subsequent half-life duration would bring about one-half of the remaining effect. It would then take approximately 5 half-live (approximately 5 weeks) to realize nearly 95% of the new steady state response. Thus, assessing the training response before at least 5-6 weeks, after achieving a full training program, will always tend to underestimate the true magnitude of the biochemical change within the working muscles. This illustrates the need for the training duration to be sufficiently prolonged for the adaptive change to fully develop.

The first-order nature of this process raises an important aspect with regard to detraining. If training is stopped, for even a brief period of time, a significant regression of the increase in mitochondrial content can occur (51-54). Again, the change in mitochondrial content will be non-linear over time. For example, in the first week (i.e., first half-life) of detraining, the elevated mitochondrial content will decline approximately 50% of the way toward the lower non-trained value (Figure 1). Further, the second and subsequent weeks of detraining will permit additional declines in mitochondrial content, each representing one-half of the remaining fall toward the normal pretraining value. Thus, because of the first-order nature of protein turnover, the greatest absolute change in the detraining process occurs initially. This indicates that the exercise program should be routinely performed, if the peak adaptive response is to be maintained. Hickson (55) has shown that training induced biochemical changes in muscle can be optimized by running almost daily (i.e., 6 days/week). This is consistent with the need to maintain the training stimulus operant within the muscle continuously over time. As discussed by Booth (56), if a one week period of detraining has occurred, a disproportional duration of training would be necessary for the mitochondrial content to recover fully, even if the full training schedule is quickly reestablished (Figure 1). Recall that during the adaptive process each week of training permits only one-half of the change possible. Thus, approximately 4 weeks would be required to permit full recovery of the mitochondrial content. Although this extended period of time would be needed to recover from the initial decline in mitochondrial content, the recovery of other training responses, such as altered blood triglyceride content (57), may follow a very different time course. Therefore, as discussed below, the existence of relatively small differences in mitochondrial content may have little impact on the recovery of exercise performance following a brief period of inactivity.

Exercise Intensity. The importance of exercise intensity was first apparent when comparing the response induced by swimming versus treadmill running training programs. Swim training does not produce as great an increase in mitochondrial content in animals as found with running (10,58). In fact, early studies evaluating an exercise response with swim training failed to find a significant biochemical change in the hindlimb muscles (59). It is likely that the weight-bearing activity associated with treadmill running exaggerates the celluar stimulus required to induce a large biochemical response. In general, the greater the exercise intensity the greater will be the induced response within the working muscles (44,60,61). This generalization, however, must be tempered by the known ordered pattern of muscle fiber type recruitment mentioned above (44). This becomes evident from the data presented in Figure 2, showing the increase in cytochrome c content (an index of mitochondrial content) in the three fiber types as a function of intensity of treadmill running. This figure was generated after first determining the influence of increasing daily duration of exercise, for training programs at each running intensity (10, 20, 30, 40, 50, and 60 meters/minute) (44). The peak response obtained for each running intensity, which usually corresponded to an asymptotic value, was then plotted against exercise intensity. This provides a characterization of the intensity influence that is essentially independent of the duration of daily exercise (44).

It is apparent that the fast-twitch red fiber section of the vastus lateralis and the slow-twitch red soleus muscles adapt with a nearly linear increase in mitochondrial content over the easy-to-moderate range of exercise conditions (10, 20, and 30 m/min). This response emphasizes the importance of exercise intensity in inducing the biochemical change. Indeed, there is a relatively large adaptive change with only small changes in exercise intensity as reflected in treadmill speed. However, it is obvious that the increase in mitochondrial content, that occurs with increasing treadmill speed, is not linear. In the case of the fast-twitch red muscle section, a maximal response was found with training after speeds of approximately 30 m/min (Figure 2). This corresponds to an estimated exercise intensity for the rat of approximately 80 - 85% of its maximal oxygen consumption (62). The brief proportional response phase up to 30 m/min, together with the plateau, could account for the apparent lack of an intensity effect observed in some studies (61). Although this plateau suggests that exercise intensity is no longer important, a more physiological interpretation seems appropriate. It may be that this fiber type was recruited in an increasing manner over the lower speeds, but that a saturation of this motor unit pool occurred at approximately 30 - 40 m/min. If this were the case, then treadmill running at speeds of 50 and 60 m/min could not be accomplished without the involvement of additional motor units. These additional motor units may be the fast-twitch white fibers. There was no change in cytochrome c content in the fast-twitch white section throughout the mild to moderate exercise intensity. However, an adaptive change became apparent in the fast-twitch white section with increasing exercise intensity above 30 - 40 m/min (Figure 2). This corresponds to the

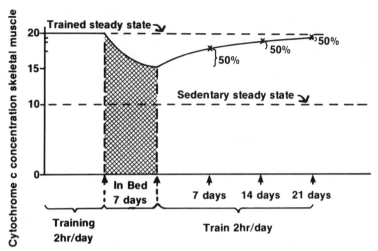

Figure 1. The predicted consequences of one week of detraining and the time of retraining required to recover the full increase in cytochrome c content (an index of mitochondrial content) in the working muscle. Note that in one week of inactivity (approx. 1 half-life), nearly 50% of the training effect is lost. Similarly, each week of retraining recovers approx. 50% of the way toward the full training effect. Since the process exhibits first-order kinetics, it takes longer to recover fully. "Reproduced with permission from Ref. 56. Copyright 1977, 'New York Academy of Sciences'."

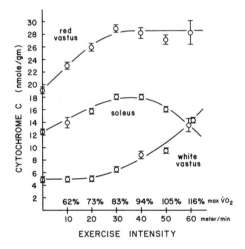

Figure 2. The influence of exercise intensity (treadmill running) on muscle cytochrome c content in the rat. Red vastus = fast-twitch red fiber section; Soleus = slow-twitch red fiber section; White vastus = fast-twitch white fiber section. "Reproduced with permission from Ref. 44. Copyright 1982, 'American Physiological Society'."

treadmill speeds where the response in the fast-twitch red section reached a plateau. Thus, the general response to training intensity, illustrated in Figure 2, is consistent with the expected ordered pattern of motor unit recruitment. These data also illustrate that care must be exercised when interpreting the training response obtained from mixed muscle sections, where each component fiber type may be adapting in a quantitatively different manner. Nonetheless, it is clear that the intensity of exercise exerts a profound influence on the magnitude of the biochemical change. Further, this response need not be similar for all fiber types. For example, at the most intense training program of 60 m/min, the cytochrome c content in the fast-twitch white fiber section was 3.0-fold normal, but only 1.5-fold normal in the fast-twitch red muscle section. This quantitative difference may be expected, if the stimulus inducing the increase in oxidative capacity is at all influenced by the preexisting mitochondrial content within the muscle fiber. Note that the cytochrome c content in the fast-twitch red section is approximately 4-times that of the fast-twitch white section (see y-axis of Figure 2). Thus, it is probable that a greater training stimulus is needed to bring about an adaptation in the well-endowed high-oxidative fibers as compared with the low-oxidative fibers. This is consistent with the general impression concerning training adaptations. Individuals who possess a relatively high aerobic work capacity must train "harder" in order to achieve a significant adaptive change (63).

Exercise Bout Duration. The general expectation that training programs which require longer daily exercise bouts produce greater adaptations has been found for the biochemical changes in muscle (44,60,64). Although lengthening exercise bout duration appears to induce a fairly linear increase in mitochondrial content (44,60,64), there is probably a finite range for this relationship. When exercise duration was very prolonged (i.e., 4 hr/day), the adaptive change was not different from that found when daily exercise involved running 2 hr/day (60). Thus, there is an exercise bout duration which, when exceeded, does not produce any added increase in mitochondrial content. Further, it is probable that the relationship between the biochemical adaptation in muscle and exercise bout duration can be described as a first order process where the influence of time is not constant (44). This is illustrated in Figure 3 for the increase in cytochrome c content in the fast-twitch white muscle section of trained rats. This relationship indicates that, during steady state training, the initial minutes of the exercise bout are the most important in creating the cellular stimulus that induces the biochemical change. The further increase in this cellular stimulus diminishes as the duration of each exercise bout increases, until an exercise bout duration is reached where added time has little if any impact. Although little is known about the exact signal within the cell that produces the increase in mitochondrial content, it may be in some way influenced by the existing oxidative capacity of the muscle fiber. For example, the decreasing importance of exercise bout duration could be explained if the magnitude of the cellular stimulus were modified by the adaptive response itself. Thus, the third 15 minute period of exercise would be expected to induce a smaller effect than the first

15 minute period of exercise, since there already exists a significant adaptive response caused by the initial exercise time period.
Another example may be the exaggerated increase in mitochondrial
content in the low oxidative fast-twitch white section, as compared
to the high oxidative fast-twitch red section, during intense
exercise training. However, unlike a simple change in exercise bout
duration, it is not known whether the utilization of each muscle
type was the same during the intense exercise bouts.

Interaction Between Exercise Duration and Intensity.   Although
exercise bout duration and intensity are distinct training parameters, they also interact to further alter the adaptive response.
This becomes apparent when noting the time necessary to achieve the
maximal adaptive change for each of the running intensities.   This
is best illustrated by the response in the fast-twitch white muscle
(Figure 3). The greater the intensity of exercise, the more rapidy
the change in cytochrome c content approaches its peak asymptotic
response. Thus, it is possible to achieve the same adaptive change
within muscle running for a shorter time/day, if the intensity of
exercise is increased accordingly. The factor(s) that change(s)
within the muscle cell enabling the initial minutes of exercise to
produce a greater training stimulus is not known. However, the
exaggerated metabolic response that occurs within muscle as exercise
intensity is increased may be implicated. Thus, exercise intensity
affects both the magnitude of the adaptive response, as well as the
exercise bout time necessary to achieve the peak response.

Functional Significance of Training Adaptations in Muscle

The increase in mitochondrial content within trained muscle could
have several significant functional influences during exercise.
First, the greater biochemical capacity for ATP provision via
aerobic metabolism could greatly increase the maximal oxygen consumption of muscle. This would be true if a) muscle could utilize a
greater ATP turnover than evident at maximal aerobic work capacity
prior to training, and b) the greater mitochondrial content was
supplied with sufficient oxygen to support the greater ATP turnover.
Since muscle exhibits a depletion of phosphocreatine (PCr) and, at
times, a reduction in ATP content during severe contraction conditions (37,39,65,66), it is probable that a higher energy utilization
could have occurred if more energy were available to meet the
demand. Thus, the potential that an increased mitochondrial content
might increase the maximal oxygen consumption of muscle probably
rests on the availability of oxygen. An increased supply of oxygen
to mitochondria of contracting muscle would occur if a) there was an
increased extraction of oxygen from the arterial blood flowing
through the muscle, and/or b) there was a greater blood flow through
the muscle (arterial blood oxygen content remains remarkably constant during all intensities of exercise (67). Oxygen extraction
across working muscle during maximal exercise is generally very
large (approximately 80% or more), even in untrained individuals
(67). A small increase in oxygen extraction (approximately 10-15%)
across working muscle after training has been observed (63,68), but
not consistently (25,69). Thus, an increase in oxygen supply due to
a greater extraction could not possibly support all of the large

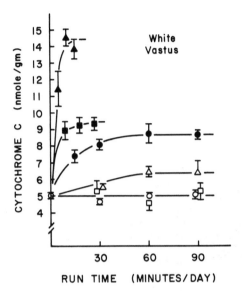

Figure 3.   The influence of exercise duration, during different intensities of treadmill running, on cytochrome c content in the white section of the vastus lateralis muscle (fast-twitch white fibers) of rats.   Running speed: (O) 10 m/min, (□) 20 m/min, (△) 30 m/min, (●) 40 m/min, (■) 50 m/min, (▲) 60 m/min. "Reproduced with permission from Ref. 44.   Copyright 1982, 'American Physiological Society'."

increase in mitochondrial content (e.g., 100%) typically found with
endurance training. This indicates that blood flow must be increased if the greater capacity for oxidative metabolism within the
trained muscle is to be utilized maximally. Measurements evaluating
the potential for changes in peak blood flow during maximal exercise
have provided equivocal results (70). Thus, there is little
assurance that training greatly alters maximal blood flow. Recent
evidence, obtained in trained rats using radiolabeled microspheres,
has demonstrated a significant increase in peak muscle blood flow in
muscle of trained rats (71). However, the increase of approximately
40 - 50% was found only in the low oxidative fast-twitch white
muscle fiber section. Although this appears to be a significant
change, its overall contribution to an increase in total body oxygen
consumption of the animal would be rather small. This low mitochondrial fiber section receives only approximately 20 - 25% of the
blood flow delivered to the high oxidative fast-twitch red section
(32,33). Therefore, the red muscle fiber types probably account for
at least 80% of the maximal oxygen consumption of the rat (33).
This religates any change in peak blood flow to the fast-twitch
white section due to training as exerting a relatively minor
influence on total body maximal oxygen consumption. Similarly, in
humans, training induces a change in maximal oxygen consumption that
is relatively small (e.g., typically 15 - 25%), compared to the
increase in mitochondrial content induced in the working muscle
(e.g., 54). Thus, it is generally recognized that the full potential of the enhanced oxidative capacity is not fully realized.

Davies, et al (72) recently reported interesting data which
illustrate the relationship between oxygen transport capacity and
maximal oxygen consumption during exercise. They found, as expected, that reducing the oxygen transport capacity by decreasing
hemoglobin concentration with an iron deficient diet, greatly
decreased the maximal oxygen consumption during exercise in rats.
During the subsequent iron refeeding period, the time course of the
return of maximal oxygen consumption nicely corresponded to the time
course of the recovery of oxygen transport capacity (i.e., hemoglobin content). Further, when the oxygen transport capacity of iron
deficient rats was returned to normal by infusion of packed red
blood cells, the maximal oxygen consumption during exercise essentially recovered to normal (73). These results illustrate the
general finding that maximal aerobic work capacity is closely
related to maximal cardiovascular transport of oxygen (74). Therefore, the functional significance of the adaptive increase in mitochondrial content may be related to cellular responses within the
working muscle during submaximal exercise. Oxygen transport is
discussed in more detail in the Trace Element chapter by McDonald
and Saltman.

Cellular Responses in Trained Muscle. Recent evidence, obtained
from appropriate measurements of metabolites within the cell during
contractions, suggests that skeletal muscle of trained individuals
is better able to adjust, as compared to skeletal muscle of untrained individuals, to the energy demands of a submaximal contraction effort. This is apparent since metabolic conditions altered by
contractions within trained muscle change less than in untrained
muscle from that found at rest. For example, the PCr content of

muscle decreases in proportion to exercise intensity throughout the submaximal range of exercise (66,75). During moderately intense contraction conditions, the decrease in PCr content to trained muscle of rats is less than that of untrained muscle (40). Similarly, the decrease in PCr content during submaximal cycle exercise (150 watts) in humans was less after physical training (76). Thus, a greater work output (i.e., energy turnover) can be achieved after training for the same decrease in PCr concentration.

The decrease in PCr, through the cell's corresponding increase in inorganic phosphate concentration (77), is thought to contribute to the cellular signal that stimulates the mitochondria to increase respiration (78,79). This could be part of the response that accounts for the tight coupling between mitochondrial ATP production (and, therefore, oxygen consumption) and the greater energy demands as exercise intensity increases. If the decrease in PCr contributes to the cellular signal to accelerate mitochondrial respiration (78,79), then a higher rate of oxygen consumption seems to occur at a relatively smaller intracellular signal driving mitochondrial respiration. This is reasonable since there are more mitochondria within the trained muscle fiber to respond and rephosphorylate ADP to ATP (5,23). Thus, trained muscle seems to be able to function at a given oxygen consumption (work rate) with a smaller metabolic signal driving mitochondrial respiration; alternatively, trained muscle can function at a higher oxygen consumption (i.e., work rate) at the same apparent cellular stimulus as found in untrained muscle working at a lower oxygen consumption. Thus, it is probable that the training induced change in mitochondrial content alters metabolic control parameters.

Another influence of the training adaptation may be during the transition from resting metabolism to the accelerated rate of respiration required by contractions. For example, a higher mitochondrial density within trained muscle might effect a more rapid transition toward a steady state aerobic energy provision at the onset of contractions. If the energy demands were being better met by mitochondrial respiration, then the rate of anaerobic energy production could be less. That this occurs is suggested by the cellular content of lactic acid that develops at the onset of contractions (40). Lactate content increased to 13.2 ± 1.31 μmole/g in fast-twitch red muscle of sedentary animals compared to only 7.1 ± 0.84 in trained muscle during the first minute of contractions (40). These results are typical (25,76,80) and could represent the favored metabolic situation in trained muscle that contributes to a more rapid achievement of steady state oxygen consumption (81,82,83) and a reduced circulating lactate content (76,80) observed after exercise training.

Altered Substrate Utilization by Trained Muscle. It is likely that the greater mitochondrial content also serves to alter the energy substrate utilized during prolonged submaximal exercise. This probably contributes to the much enhanced endurance performance typical of the endurance trained individual. It has long been recognized that trained individuals obtain a greater fraction of their energy needs from the oxidation of fatty acids than untrained individuals exercising at the same work intensity (cf. 6). The greater extent of lipid oxidation, evident by a lower respiratory quotient of trained individuals, has been confirmed by direct measurements of enhanced $^{14}CO_2$ production from infused labeled palmitate (84). Although an enhanced concentration of circulating fatty acids can increase fat oxidation and extend exercise time (85,86), the increased lipid oxidation in trained individuals is apparent even when circulating fatty acid levels are not different from that of the non-trained (87). Thus, there is probably some fundamental alteration within the working muscle to permit the greater rate of beta oxidation. Recall that an increase in the capacity for fatty acid oxidation is included in the adaptive response of a greater mitochondrial content (15). A greater enzyme content within the muscle could result in a greater rate of fatty acid oxidation, even when the same fatty acid concentration is available for beta oxidation (15). One direct consequence of obtaining a greater fraction of the energy from fatty acid derived acetylCoA is to lessen the demand for other carbon sources for oxidation. This would be expected to reduce the rate of glycolysis and potentially the rate of glycogen utilization in the working muscle. Recent evidence indicates that enhancing fatty acid oxidation does, indeed, spare muscle glycogen (85,86,88). These metabolic changes are discussed in more detail in the following chapter by Goodman. Since the depletion of muscle glycogen stores during prolonged submaximal exercise corresponds with exhaustion, there is now reason to couple the training adaptation of an increased mitochondrial content within the working muscle to the marked increase in endurance performance. Specifically, the greater mitochondrial content permits an enhanced energy supply from lipid oxidation; this, in turn, retards the rate of utilization of muscle glycogen, thereby permitting muscle glycogen to be used over an extended exercise time. Although many other physiological, metabolic and endocrine changes must be important in the training process, biochemical adaptations within the working muscles appear to exert a significant influence on energy metabolism and muscle performance.

Summary

Routinely performed physical activity, such as cycling or running, increases one's endurance capacity for prolonged submaximal work. Associated with this response are biochemical changes within the working muscles. This includes an increase in the content of mitochondria, the cellular organelle where energy (ATP) is produced by the oxidation of fuels (glucose and fat) in the presence of oxygen. The magnitude of this increase in mitochondrial content is influenced, in a complex manner, by the intensity and duration of exercise, since not all skeletal muscle fibers may be recruited and there are marked differences between muscle fiber types. Most mammalian muscle is composed of three different fiber types: 1) slow-twitch red (Type I) which is relatively slow contracting and has a high mitochondrial content and endurance capacity, 2) fast-twitch red (Type IIa) which is relatively fast contracting and has a high mitochondrial content and endurance capacity, and 3) fast-twitch white (Type IIb) which is relatively fast contracting and has a low mitochondrial content and endurance capacity. These fiber types are recruited progressively beginning with Type I, then Type

IIa and finally Type IIb as the intensity of exercise increases. Thus, regular physical activity of moderate intensity will increase the mitochondrial content of primarily Type I and Type IIa fibers, while proportionally larger increases are induced in Type IIb fibers during more intense physical training when these fibers are recruited. One major benefit of enhancing the mitochondrial content in the working muscles is related to the much greater capacity of the muscle to oxidize fat for energy. A greater supply of energy from fat serves to preserve the intramuscular glucose store (glycogen) which is in limited supply. Depletion of muscle glycogen has been implicated as a factor causing fatigue during prolonged moderately intense exercise (e.g., running for more than 1 hr). Thus, the enhanced mitochondrial content and its related increase in fat oxidation probably contribute to the greatly improved endurance performance following exercise training.

Acknowledgments

Cited work by the authors was supported by National Institutes of Health Grant AM-21617 and Research Career Development Award AM-00681 (to R.L.T.).

Literature Cited

1. Lawrie, R. A. (1953) The activity of the cytochrome system in muscle and its relation to myoglobin. Biochem. J. 55: 298-305.
2. Lawrie, R. A. (1953) Effect of enforced exercise on myoglobin concentration in muscle. Nature London. 171: 1069-71.
3. John-Alder, H. (1984) Seasonal variations in activity, aerobic energetic capacities, and plasma thyroid hormones (T3 and T4) in an iguanid lizard. J. Comp. Physiol. B. 154: 409-419.
4. Armstrong, R. B., Ianuzzo, C. D., Kunz, T. H. (1977) Histochemical and biochemical properties of flight muscle fibers in the little brown, bat, Myotis lucifugus. J. Comp. Physiol. 119: 141-54.
5. Holloszy, J. O. (1973) Biochemical adaptations to exercise: aerobic metabolism. Ex. Sport. Sci. Rev. 1: 45-71.
6. Holloszy, J. O. and Booth, F. W. (1976) Biochemical adaptations to endurance exercise in muscle. Ann. Rev. Physiol. 38: 273-291, 1976.
7. Saltin, B. and Gollnick, P.D. (1983) Skeletal muscle adaptability: significance for metabolism and performance. In Handbook of Physiology, Section 10: Skeletal Muscle (Peachey, L. D., ed.), pp. 555-631, Am. Physiol. Soc., Bethesda, MD.
8. Holloszy, J. O. and Coyle, E. F. (1984) Adaptations of skeletal muscle to endurance exercise and their metabolic consequences. J. Appl. Physiol.: Respirat. Environ. Exercise Physiol. 56: 831-8.
9. Salmons, S. and Henriksson, J. (1981) The adaptive response of skeletal muscle to increased use. Muscle Nerve 4: 94-105.
10. Holloszy, J. O. (1967) Biochemical adaptations in muscle. Effects of exercise on mitochondrial oxygen uptake and respiratory enzyme activity in skeletal muscle. J. Biol. Chem. 242: 2278-82.

11. Saltin, B., Henriksson, J., Nygaard, E., Andersen, P. and
     Jansson, E. (1977) Fiber types and metabolic potentials of
     skeletal muscles in sedentary man and endurance runners. In
     The Marathon: Physiological, Medical, Epidemiological and
     Psychological Studies (Milvy, P., ed), pp. 3-29, Annals of the
     New York Academy of Sciences, Vol. 301, New York, NY.
12. Gollnick, P.D., Ianuzzo, C. D. and King, D.W. (1971) Ultra-
     structural and enzyme changes in muscles with exercise. In
     Muscle Metabolism During Exercise (Pernow, B. and Saltin, B.,
     eds), pp. 69-85, Advances in Experimental Medicine and Biology,
     Vol. 11, Plenum Press, New York, NY.
13. Morgan, T. E., Cobb, L. A., Short, F. A., Ross, R. and Gunn, D.
     R. (1971) Effects of long term exercise on human muscle
     mitochndria. In Muscle Metabolism During Exercise (Pernow, B.
     and Saltin, B., eds), pp. 87-95, Advances in Experimental
     Medicine and Biology, Vol. 11, Plenum Press, New York, NY.
14. Baldwin, K. M., Klinkerfuss, G. H., Terjung, R. L., Molé, P. A.
     and Holloszy, J. O. (1972) Respiratory capacity of white, red,
     and intermediate muscle: adaptive response to exercise. Am. J.
     Physiol. 222: 373-8.
15. Molé, P. A., Oscai, L. B. and Holloszy, J. O. (1971) Adaptation
     of muscle to exercise. Increase in levels of palmityl CoA
     synthetase, carnitine palmityl-transferase and palmityl CoA
     dehydrogenase and in the capacity to oxidize fatty acids. J.
     Clin. Invest. 50: 2323-30.
16. Costill, D. L., Fink, W. J., Getchell, L. H., Ivy, J. L. and
     Witzmann, F. A. (1979) Lipid metabolism in skeletal muscle of
     endurance trained males and females. J. Appl. Physiol.:
     Respirat. Environ. Exercise Physiol. 47: 787-91.
17. Winder, W. W., Baldwin, K. M. and Holloszy, J. O. (1975)
     Exercise-induced increase in the capacity of rat skeletal
     muscle to oxidize ketones. Can. J. Physiol. Pharmacol. 53:
     86-91.
18. Holloszy, J. O., Oscai, L. B., Don, I. J. and Molé, P.A. (1970)
     Mitochondrial citric acid cycle and related enzymes: adaptive
     response to exercise. Biochem. Biophys. Res. Commun. 40:
     1368-73.
19. Holloszy, J. O., Booth, F. W., Winder, W. W. and Fitts, R. H.
     (1975) Biochemical adaptation of skeletal muscle to prolonged
     physical exercise. In Metabolic Adaptation to Prolonged
     Physical Exercise (Howald, H. and Poortmans, J. R., eds.), pp.
     438-47, Birkhauser Verlag, Basel.
20. Wittenberg, B. A., Wittenberg, J. B. and Caldwell, P.R.B.
     (1975) Role of myoglobin in the oxygen supply to red skeletal
     muscle. J. Biol. Chem. 250: 9038-43.
21. Cole, R. P. (1982) Myoglobin function in exercising skeletal
     muscle. Science 216: 523-525.
22. Pattengale, P. K. and Holloszy, J. O. (1967) Augmentation of
     skeletal muscle myoglobin by a program of treadmill running.
     Am. J. Physiol. 213: 783-5.
23. Gollnick, P. D. and Saltin, B. (1982) Significance of skeletal
     muscle oxidative enzyme enhancement with endurance training.
     Clin. Physiol. 2: 1-12.

24. Winder, W. W., Baldwin, K. M. and Holloszy, J. O. (1974) Enzymes involved in ketone utilization in different types of muscle: adaptation to exercise. Eur. J. Biochem. 47: 461-7.

25. Saltin, B., Nazar, K., Costill, D. L., Stein, E., Jansson, E., Essen, B. and Gollnick, P.D. (1976) The nature of the training response; peripheral and central adaptations to one-legged exercise. Acta Physiol. Scand. 96: 289-305.

26. Burke, R. E. (1981) Motor units: anatomy, physiology, and functional organization. In Handbook of Physiology: The Nervous System 2 (Brookhart, J. M. and Mountcastle, V. B., eds.), pp. 345-422, Am. Physiol. Soc., Bethesda, MD.

27. Close, R. I. (1972) Dynamic properties of mammalian skeletal muscles. Physiol. Rev. 52: 129-197.

28. Baldwin, K. M., Winder, W. W. and Holloszy, J. O. (1975) Adaptation of actomyosin ATPase in different types of muscle to endurance exercise. Am. J. Physiol. 229: 422-6.

29. Martonosi, A. N. and Beeler, T. J. (1983) Mechanism of Ca^{2+} transport by sarcoplasmic reticulum. In Handbook of Physiology: Skeletal Muscle (Peachey, L. D., ed.), pp. 417-485, Am. Physiol. Soc., Bethesda, MD.

30. Barany, M. (1967) ATPase activity of myosin correlated with speed of muscle shortening. J. Gen. Physiol. 50, Suppl. pt. 2: 197-218.

31. Brooke, M. H. and Kaiser, K. K. (1970) Three myosin adenosine triphosphatase systems: the nature of their pH lability and sulfhydryl dependence. J. Histochem. Cytochem. 18: 670-2.

32. Laughlin, M. H. and Armstrong, R. B. (1982) Muscular blood flow distribution patterns as a function of running speed in rats. Am. J. Physiol. 243: H296-H306.

33. Mackie, B. G. and Terjung, R. L. (1983) Blood flow to different skeletal muscle fiber types during contraction. Am. J. Physiol. 245: H265-H275.

34. Baldwin, K. M., Winder, W. W., Terjung, R. L. and Holloszy, J. O. (1973) Glycolytic enzymes in different types of skeletal muscles: adaptation to exercise. Am. J. Physiol. 225: 962-6.

35. Hintz, C. S., Lowry, C. V., Kaiser, K. K., McKee, D. and Lowry, O. H. (1980) Enzyme levels in individual rat muscle fibers. Am. J. Physiol. 239: C58-C65.

36. Burke, R. E., Levine, D. N., Zajac, F. E., Tsairis, P. and Engel, W. K. (1971) Mammalian motor units: physiological-histo-chemical correlation in three types of cat gastrocnemius. Science 174: 709-12.

37. Meyer, R. A. and Terjung, R. L. (1979) Differences in ammonia and adenylate metabolism in contracting fast and slow muscle. Am. J. Physiol. 237: C111-C118.

38. Rall, J. (1985) Energetic aspects of skeletal muscle contraction: implications of fiber types. Ex. Sport. Sci. Rev. Vol. 13.

39. Meyer, R. A., Dudley, G. A. and Terjung, R. L. (1980) Ammonia and IMP in different skeletal muscle fibers after exercise in rats. J. Appl. Physiol.: Respirat. Environ. Exercise Physiol. 49: 1037-41.

40. Dudley, G. A. and Terjung, R. L. (1985) Influence of aerobic metabolism on IMP accumulation in fast-twitch muscle. Am. J. Physiol. 248: C37-C42.

58. Baldwin, K. M., Fitts, R. H., Booth, F. W., Winder, W. W. and
     Holloszy, J. O. (1975) Depletion of muscle and liver glycogen
     during exercise. Pflugers Arch. 354: 203-12.
59. Hearn, G. R. and Wainio, W. W. (1956) Succinic dehydrogenase
     activity of the heart and skeletal muscle of exercise rats.
     Am. J. Physiol. 185: 348-50.
60. Terjung, R. L. (1976) Muscle fiber involvement during training
     of different intensities and durations. Am. J. Physiol. 230:
     946-50.
61. Harms, S. J. and Hickson, R. C. (1983) Skeletal muscle
     mitochondria and myoglobin, endurance, and intensity of
     training. J. Appl. Physiol.: Respirat. Environ. Exercise
     Physiol. 54: 798-802.
62. Shepherd, R. E. and Gollnick, P. D. (1976) Oxygen uptake of
     rats at different work intensities. Pflugers Arch. 362:
     219-22.
63. Saltin, B., Blomqvist, G., Mitchell, J. H., Johnson, R. L.,
     Wildenthal, K. and Chapman, C. B. (1968) Response to exercise
     after bed rest and after training. Circulation 38, Suppl. 7:
     1-78.
64. Fitts, R. H., Booth, F. W., Winder, W. W. and Holloszy, J. O.
     (1975) Skeletal muscle respiratory capacity, endurance, and
     glycogen utilization. Am. J. Physiol. 228: 1029-33.
65. Sahlin, K., Palmskog, G. and Hultman, E. (1978) Adenine
     nucleotide and IMP contents of the quadriceps muscle in man
     after exercise. Pflugers Arch. 374: 193-8.
66. Karlsson, J. (1971) Lactate and phosphagen concentrations in
     working muscle of man. Acta Physiol. Scand. Suppl. 358: 1-72.
67. Astrand, P.-O. and Rodahl, K. (1977) Textbook of Work
     Physiology, pp. 182-4, McGraw-Hill, Inc., New York, NY.
68. Ekblom, B., Astrand, P.-O., Saltin, B., Stenberg, J. and
     Wallstrom, B. (1968) Effect of training on the circulatory
     response to exercise. J. Appl. Physiol. 24: 518-28.
69. Kilborn, A. and Astrand, I. (1971) Physical training with
     submaximal intensities in women. II. Effect on cardiac output.
     Scand. J. Clin. Lab. Invest. 28: 163-75.
70. Hudlicka, O. (1977) Effect of training on macro- and
     microcirculatory changes in exercise. Ex. Sport. Sci. Rev. 5:
     181-230.
71. Mackie, B. G. and Terjung, R. L. (1983) Influence of training
     on blood flow to different skeletal muscle fiber types. J.
     Appl. Physiol.: Respirat. Environ. Exercise Physiol. 55:
     1072-8.
72. Davies, K. J. A., Maguire, J. J., Brooks, G. A., Dallman, P.
     R. and Packer, L. (1982) Muscle mitochondrial bioenergetics,
     oxygen supply, and work capacity during dietary iron deficiency
     and repletion. Am. J. Physiol. 242: E418-E427.
73. Davies, K. J. A., Donovan, C. M., Refino, C. J., Brooks, G. A.,
     Packer, L. and Dallman, P. R. (1984) Distinguishing effects of
     anemia and muscle iron deficiency on exercise bioenergetics in
     the rat. Am. J. Physiol. 246: E535-E543.
74. Gledhill, N. (1985) The influence of altered blood volume and
     oxygen transport capacity on aerobic performance. Ex. Sport.
     Sci. Rev. Vol. 13.

41. Dudley, G. A. and Terjung, R. L. (1985) Influence of acidosis on AMP deaminase activity in contracting fast-twitch muscle. Am. J. Physiol. 248: C43-C50.

42. Walmsley, B., Hodgson, J. A. and Burke, R. E. (1978) Forces produced by medial gastrocnemius and soleus muscles during locomotion in freely moving cats. J. Neurophysiol. 41: 1203-15.

43. Sullivan, T. E. and Armstrong, R. B. (1978) Rat locomotory muscle fiber activity during trotting and galloping. J. Appl. Physiol.: Respirat. Environ. Exercise Physiol. 44: 358-63.

44. Dudley, G. A., Abraham, W. M. and Terjung, R. L. (1982) Influence of exercise intensity and duration on biochemical adaptations in skeletal muscle. J. Appl. Physiol.: Respirat. Environ. Exercise Physiol. 53: 844-50.

45. Burke, R. E. and Edgerton, V. R. (1975) Motor unit properties and selective involvement in movement. Ex. Sport. Sci. Rev. 3: 31-81.

46. Ariano, M. A., Armstrong, R. B. and Edgerton, V. R. (1973) Hindlimb muscle fiber populations of five mammals. J. Histochem. Cytochem. 21: 51-55.

47. Armstrong, R. B. and Phelps, R. O. (1984) Muscle fiber type composition of the rat hindlimb. Am. J. Anatomy 171: 259-72.

48. Costill, D. L., Daniels, J., Evans, W., Fink, W., Krahenbuhl, G. and Saltin, B. (1976) Skeletal muscle enzymes and fiber composition in male and female track athletes. J. Appl. Physiol. 40: 149-54.

49. Lowry, C. V., Kimmey, J. S., Felder, S., Chi, M.-Y., Kaiser, K. K., Passonneau, P. N., Kirk, K. A. and Lowry, O. H. (1978) Enzyme patterns in single human muscle fibers. J. Biol. Chem. 253: 8269-77.

50. Schimke, R. T. and Doyle, D. (1970) Control of enzyme levels in animals tissues. Ann. Rev. Biochem. 39: 929-76.

51. Terjung, R. L. (1979) The turnover of cytochrome c in different skeletal muscle fiber types of the rat. Biochem. J. 178: 569-74.

52. Terjung, R. L. (1975) Cytochrome c turnover in skeletal muscle. Biochem. Biophys. Res. Commun. 66: 173-8.

53. Booth, F. W. and Holloszy, J. O. (1977) Cytochrome c turnover in rat skeletal muscles. J. Biol. Chem. 252: 416-19.

54. Henriksson, J. and Reitman, J. S. (1977) Time course of changes in human skeletal muscle succinate dehydrogenase and cytochrome oxidase activities and maximal oxygen uptake with physical activity and inactivity. Acta Physiol. Scand. 99: 91-7.

55. Hickson, R. C. (1981) Skeletal muscle cytochrome c and myoglobin, endurance, and frequency of training. J. Appl. Physiol.: Respirat. Environ. Exercise Physiol. 51: 746-9, 1981.

56. Booth, F. W. (1977) Effects of endurance exercise on cytochrome c turnover in skeletal muscle. In The Marathon: Physiological, Medical, Epidemiological, and Psychological Studies (Milvy, P., ed.), pp. 431-439, Annals of the New York Academy of Sciences, Vol. 301, New York, NY.

57. Oscai, L. B., Patterson, J. A., Bogard, E. L., Beck, R. J. and Rothermel, B. L. (1972) Normalization of serum triglycerides and lipoprotein electrophoretic patterns by exercise. Am. J. Cardiol. 30: 775-80.

75. Bergstrom, J., Harris, R. C., Hultman, E. and Nordesjö, L. O. (1971) Energy rich phosphagens in dynamic and static work. In Muscle Metabolism During Exercise (Pernow, B. and Saltin, B., eds.), pp. 341-55, Advances in Experimental Medicine and Biology, Vol. 11, Plenum Press, New York, NY.

76. Karlsson, J., Nordesjö, L.-O., Jorfeldt; L. and Saltin, B. (1972) Muscle lactate, ATP, and CP levels during exercise after physical training in man. J. Appl. Physiol. 33: 199-203.

77. Meyer, R. A., Sweeney, H. L. and Kushmerick, M. J. (1984) A simple analysis of the "phosphocreatine shuttle". Am. J. Physiol. 246: C365-77, 1984.

78. Erecinska, M., Wilson, D. F. and Nishiki, K. (1978) Homeostatic regulation of cellular energy metabolism: experimental characterization in vivo and fit to a model. Am. J. Physiol. 234: C82-C89, 1978.

79. Erecinska, M. and Wilson, D. F. (1982) Regulation of cellular energy metabolism. J. Memb. Biol. 70: 1-14.

80. Henriksson, J. (1977) Training induced adaptations of skeletal muscle and metabolism during submaximal exercise. J. Physiol. 270: 661-75.

81. Hickson, R. C., Bomze, H. A. and Holloszy, J. O. (1978) Faster adjustment of O_2 uptake to the energy requirement of exercise in the trained state. J. Appl. Physiol.: Respirat. Environ. Exercise Physiol. 44: 877-81.

82. Cerretelli, P., Pendergast, D., Paganelli, W. C. and Rennie, D. W. (1979) Effects of specific muscle training on VO_2 on-response and early blood lactate. J. Appl. Physiol.: Respirat. Environ. Exercise Physiol. 47: 761-9.

83. Hagberg, J. M., Hickson, R. C., Ehsani, A. A. and Holloszy, J. O. (1980) Faster adjustment to and recovery from submaximal exercise in the trained state. J. Appl. Physiol.: Respirat. Environ. Exercise Physiol. 48: 218-24.

84. Paul, P. (1971) Uptake and oxidation of substrates in the intact animal during exercise. In Muscle Metabolism During Exercise (Pernow, B. and Saltin, B., eds.), pp. 225-248, Advances in Experimental Medicine and Biology, Vol. 11, Plenum Press, New York, NY.

85. Hickson, R. C., Rennie, M. J., Conlee, R. K., Winder, W. W. and Holloszy, J. O. (1977) Effects of increased plasma free fatty acids on glycogen utilization and endurance. J. Appl. Physiol.: Respirat. Environ. Exercise Physiol. 43: 829-33.

86. Costill, D. L., Coyle, E., Dalsky, G., Evans, W., Fink, W. and Hooper, D. (1977) Effects of elevated plasma FFA and insulin on muscle glycogen usage during exercise. J. Appl. Physiol.: Respirat. Environ. Exercise Physiol. 43: 695-9.

87. Holloszy, J. O., Winder, W. W., Fitts, R. H., Rennie, M. J., Hickson, R. C. and Conlee, R. K. (1978) Energy production during exercise. In: 3rd International Symposium on Biochemistry of Exercise (Landry, F. and Orban, W. A. R., eds.), pp. 61-74, Symposia Specialists, Inc., Miami, FL.

88. Rennie, M. J., Winder, W. W. and Holloszy, J. O. (1976) A sparing effect of increased plasma free fatty acids on muscle and liver glycogen content in the exercising rat. Biochem. J. 156: 647-55.

RECEIVED May 14, 1985

Influence of Aerobic Exercise on Fuel Utilization by Skeletal Muscle

Michael N. Goodman

Department of Medicine and Physiology, Boston University School of Medicine, Boston, MA 02118

During the past decade, we have witnessed a renaissance of interest in muscular exercise and the potential benefits it may have on the health of the individual. Evidence is available that exercise can prevent or at least delay cardiovascular disease, lower risk factors for atherosclerosis, help in weight reduction and may help prevent complications of certain diseases such as diabetes (1,2). The impact physical exertion has had on our society is quite evident by the numbers of aerobic-related advertisements in non-scientific publications as well as the numbers of individuals running, walking or cycling. Years ago these activities were usually confined to the athlete, and at that time athletes may have been more concerned with what was the best foodstuff for maximum performance or endurance rather than on how physical exertion may prevent complications or delay debilitating diseases. Nevertheless, the impact of nutrition on physical performance capacity has been a subject of considerable interest for numerous years. Even today, individuals who exercise for health benefits may manipulate their diet so as to gain better performance capacity. The present review will focus on a particular aspect of this subject, specifically how the use of various metabolic fuels are regulated during muscular exercise. For the most part studies in man will be cited, but some sections will include reference to animal studies for a particular emphasis.

The question of what fuels are used by the working muscles during physical performance and the relative importance of each is not new and has been debated for a long time. Early studies as far back as 1896 suggested that carbohydrates were the only fuel that could be oxidized by the working muscles (3,4). It was only later that studies established that both carbohydrates (i.e., plasma glucose and muscle glycogen) and lipids (i.e., plasma free fatty acids and muscle triglycerides) could be utilized by the working muscles. The use of protein as a fuel also received attention in early studies, but more recent studies suggest that its usage by muscle is small in relation to carbohydrates and lipids (4).

0097–6156/86/0294–0027$06.00/0

Some insights into how carbohydrate and lipid utilization may be regulated during exercise may be gained by comparing exercise to the metabolism of starvation. As can be seen in Figure 1, exercise and starvation have several features in common. During starvation, blood glucose falls early in the fast and then remains remarkably stable. Concomittantly, circulating lipid fuels (i.e., free fatty acids and ketone bodies) rise. The fall in insulin during the fast probably orchestrates the increase in lipolysis by stimulating the breakdown of triglycerides stored in adipose tissue. Although variable glucagon may rise   early in the fast and then fall as the fast is lengthened. A somewhat similar metabolic profile occurs during exercise, especially if it is of the type that is of light to moderate intensity with a duration of one hour or longer.

Teleologically, the goal of these metabolic changes is to maintain a constant fuel supply to the brain while providing the peripheral tissues such as muscle with an alternate fuel in the form of lipid (either free fatty acids or ketone bodies) to replace glucose (5,6). As shown in Figure 2, as fasting progresses, lipid becomes the most important source of fuel for muscle, while the use of carbohydrate diminishes. This is reflected in a fall of the respiratory quotient across muscle. During exercise, carbohydrate is of prime importance as a fuel during the early minutes. As exercise progresses, lipid becomes a more important fuel. However, carbohydrate oxidation is not negligible and seems important in preventing exhaustion. In elite ultra distance runners who can remain active for 24 hours, lipid becomes the sole fuel as glycogen stores in the muscle become exhausted (7). The respiratory quotient at this time is about 0.7. These elite runners also experience a   marked reduction in power output indicating that somehow muscle glycogen may be important in maintaining maximum efficiency during exercise.

Thus, it is evident that the mobilization and provision of lipid to muscle during exercise,   like during starvation, restricts the usage of carbohydrate. If this did not occur during exercise, glycogen stores within muscle (as well as in the liver) would be depleted more rapidly than normal and may significantly limit the duration of exercise. Hypoglycemia could also result and limit performance.

Fuel reserves of the body

The importance of regulating carbohydrate stores within muscle (and liver) during aerobic work can be readily appreciated when one considers that the distance of a marathon (26.2 miles) is completed by top runners in about 130 minutes with a total energy expenditure of about 2,600 kilocalories, roughly 20 kilocalories/minute (8,9). One of the problems in completing the distance in such time is the provision of sufficient fuel to satisfy the rate of energy expenditure. As shown in Table I, the largest fuel reserve in the body is triglyceride located primarily in adipose tissue with a smaller amount in skeletal muscle. Compared to the triglyceride stores, a much smaller amount of fuel is available as glycogen stored within liver and

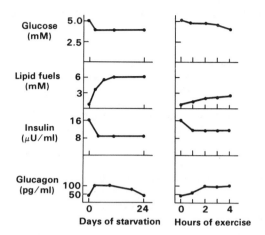

Figure 1 - Effect of starvation and exercise of moderate intensity on the concentrations of blood glucose, lipids (free fatty acids and ketone bodies), insulin and glucagon. Data from Cahill (5) and Felig and Wahren (11).

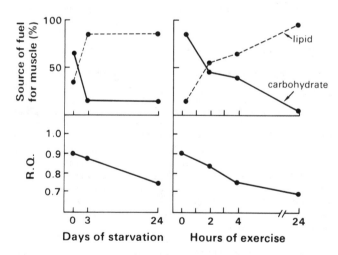

Figure 2 - Utilization of carbohydrate and lipid by skeletal muscle during starvation and exercise. Respiratory quotient (RQ) is the ratio of CO_2 produced/O_2 consumed. Data from Owen and Reichard (6), Felig and Wahren (11) and Wahren (12).

muscle. Although protein has been omitted, the caloric value of protein in the body may account for 15% of the body fuel reserves; however, its usefullness as a fuel is limited because its consumption would necessitate the dissolution of skeletal muscle.

It can be seen in Table I, that if a normal 70kg man were to undergo total starvation and remain in the basal state he could, in theory, survive for about 60 days with his fuel requirements being met by triglyceride breakdown. On the other hand, at this basal rate of metabolism, carbohydrate stores would be diminished within a day. If this individual were to run a marathon (20 kcal/min), triglyceride stores could provide energy for about 5 days, whereas, carbohydrate stores for only 90 minutes. The latter is probably an overestimation, if one considers that not all muscles would be used during the run and that the conversion of carbohydrate oxidation to ATP generation is not at 100% efficiency. With this consideration carbohydrate stores may provide energy for perhaps 60 minutes, far short of the time needed for completion of a marathon.

Factors Regulating Fuel Utilization during Aerobic Performance

From the above discussion, it is evident that the provision of fuel for the muscle is a major limiting factor during exercise and selection of fuels for oxidation by the muscle is of considerable importance in delaying the onset of fatigue, especially in the type of exertion that may go beyond 10 or 20 minutes. A number of factors can regulate fuel utilization during exercise including 1) muscle fiber type, 2) duration and intensity of exercise, 3) physical training and 4) diet.

Muscle Fiber Types.
Skeletal muscle is usually classified according to its fiber type. This classification is based upon staining properties of some muscle enzymes as well as measurement of biochemical markers (10). In man, muscle fibers are classified as being of either type I or type II (A or B) (Table II). Type I fibers are slow-twitch highly oxidative fibers with a high capillary density. These characteristics usually confer a high capability for lipid oxidation. Type II fibers on the other hand are fast-twitch fibers. Type IIA fibers are somewhat similar to those of type I in that they also have a moderately high oxidative capacity; in addition, they have a moderately high glycolytic capacity. Type IIB fibers also have a high glycolytic but low oxidative capacity.

One can usually predict from these various characteristics whether or not a particular muscle would be more involved in endurance versus sprint activity as well as the fuel or fuel mixture used. For example, as discussed in the preceding chapter by Terjung type I and IIA fibers are more involved with endurance performance relying on a fuel mixture of both lipids and carbohydrate. On the other hand, type IIB fibers are more involved with short sprint-type of activity with a fuel dependence almost exclusively on carbohydrate. The fiber composition of muscle from a few animals and man is shown in Table III. Animals raised for quick "stop and go" activity

Table I. Fuel Reserves and Rates of Utilization under Different Conditions in Humans

Tissue of source	Approximate total fuel reserve		Estimated period for which fuel store would provide energy	
	(g)	(kcal)	Days of starvation	Minutes of a marathon
Adipose tissue triglyceride	16,000	150,000	60	7143
Muscle triglyceride	200	1,800	0.72	86
Liver glycogen	90	375	0.15	18
Muscle glycogen	350	1,500	0.60	71
Blood glucose	20	80	0.03	4

Data from Newsholme (37).

Table II   Characteristics of Different Fiber Types

Characteristics	Muscle fiber type		
	I	IIA	IIB
1. Myofibrillar ATPase	slow-twitch	fast-twitch	fast-twitch
2. Mitochondrial eyzymes	high	intermediate	low
3. Glycolytic enzymes	low	intermediate	high
4. Lipids	high	intermediate	low
5. Glycogen	same	same	same
6. Capillary density	high	intermediate	low

Data from Saltin et al. (10).

Table III.   Fiber Composition of Muscle from Horses, Dogs and Man

	Percentage fiber composition	
	Type I	Type II
Horse		
Quarterhorse	7	93
Dog		
Greyhound	3	97
Man		
Untrained	53	47
Sprinters	24	76
Elite runners	79	21

Data from Newsholme and Leech (7).

(quarterhorse) or very short distance speed running (greyhound) have a high proportion of type II muscle fibers. In man, individuals considered non-athletes or untrained have an equal number of type I and II fibers, whereas, sprinters have a preponderance of type II fibers and elite distance runners more type I fibers. It is intriguing that some individuals have a high proportion (70-80%) of either type I or II fibers. It remains to be determined whether or not this is due to a genetic predisposition.

Duration and Intensity of Exercise. A key factor regulating carbohydrate as well as lipid utilization during aerobic performance is both the intensity of the exercise as well as its duration. As shown in Figure 3, the increase in glucose uptake by the working leg muscles is an early event, and the uptake is proportional to the work load (11-13). After several hours of exercise, leg glucose uptake begins to fall possibly as a result of a fall in blood glucose indicating that liver glycogen stores are nearing exhaustion. It is noteworthy that the increase in muscle glucose uptake occurs as insulin levels in plasma fall (Figure 1) indicating this response is not mediated by increased secretion of insulin (12). Whether insulin is permissive for this response remains to be determined (14). Early in the exercise, leg glucose uptake is matched by splanchnic (i.e. liver) glucose output but as liver glycogen becomes depleted splanchnic glucose output falls (11,12). Glycogen breakdown within working muscles also occurs during the early stages of exercise and its breakdown is proportional to the workload (15) (Figure 4). At high workloads (80% of VO_2 max), glycogen depletion occurs rapidly and limits duration of the exercise. Its depletion is more gradual with light to moderate exercise and may not be a limiting factor until late in the exercise. Like glycogen, muscle triglyceride breakdown can also occur during exercise (15) however, this has not been as well studied as muscle glycogen breakdown to indicate whether or not its degradation is also influenced by intensity and duration of exercise. On the other hand, it has been shown that uptake of free fatty acids from plasma by working muscle increases steadily during exercise (11,12).

From measurements of the uptake of glucose and free fatty acids and glycogen breakdown by the working muscles, one can estimate the contribution made by each fuel to the total oxidative metabolism. As shown in Table IV, during the first several hours of light to moderate exercise the majority of the fuel for the muscle is derived from plasma glucose and muscle glycogen. Between 3-4 hours, plasma free fatty acids become the more important fuel, as plasma glucose levels fall and muscle glycogen becomes depleted. Although muscle and plasma triglycerides are also utilized during exercise, their contribution to total oxidative metabolism during prolonged exercise is not precisely known since their pattern of usage throughout exercise has not been well determined. One may speculate, however, that like fatty acids their contribution to the fuel metabolism of muscle may rise as exercise is prolonged.

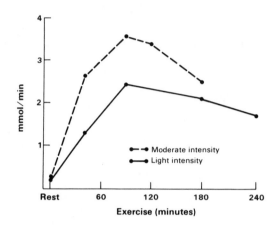

Figure 3 - **Leg glucose uptake during bicycle exercise.** Data from Wahren (12) and Wahren et al. (13).

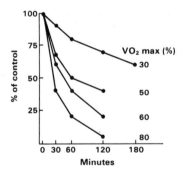

Figure 4 - Glycogen depletion from the quadraceps femoris during exercise.   Data from Essen (15).

**Table IV. Contribution of Glucose, Glycogen and Fatty Acids
to Oxygen Consumption of Leg Muscles of Man
during Mild Prolonged Exercise**

Period of exercise (minutes)	Percentage contribution to oxygen uptake		
	Muscle glycogen	Plasma glucose	Plasma fatty acids
40	36	27	37
90	22	41	37
180	14	36	50
240	8	30	62

Data from Felig and Wahren (11) and Newsholme and Leech (7). Glucose, free fatty acids and oxygen uptake and glycogen breakdown by the working muscles were determined. Calculations derived from these data assume that all substrates are completely oxidized by the working muscles. The calculations also assume that the complete metabolism of one mole of glucose (or glycogen) requires 6 moles of oxygen while one mole of fatty acid requires 25 moles of oxygen.

Physical Training. Programs of light to moderate endurance exercise (i.e. training) have been found to increase the respiratory capacity of skeletal muscle (16,17). This response is associated with both an increase in the number of mitochondria as well as amounts of oxidative enzymes. As shown in Table V, the adaptive response to training involves increases in oxidative enzyme activities in all muscle fiber types. This indicates that the major factor that determines the respiratory capacity of a muscle fiber appears to be its contractile activity; the more frequently a muscle fiber contracts the greater its mitochondrial content and oxidative capacity. In contrast to changes in mitochondrial oxidative enzymes, many of the enzymes of glycolysis either do not change or may even decrease following training (17,18). This adaptation is specific to endurance exercise since strength exercise (i.e. weight lifting) which can result in muscle hypertrophy, does not induce an increase in muscle mitochondria (8).

Due to the adaptive increase in the respiratory capacity of muscle physically trained individuals derive a greater proportion of their energy from oxidation of fat and less from carbohydrate during submaximal exercise (17,19). Ample evidence suggests that depletion of body carbohydrate stores can play an important role in the development of physical exhaustion during prolonged exercise (16,17,20). One mechanism by which training may increase endurance appears to involve a glycogen-sparing effect. Direct measurements of muscle glycogen in man and animals following submaximal exercise have shown that its content decreases more slowly following training (17,20). It is also of interest that physical training can lead to less hepatic glycogen depletion following submaximal exercise (20). The beneficial effect of this adaptation is to protect the trained individual or animal against hepatic glycogen depletion and the development of hypoglycemia during prolonged exercise.

Diet. There is a widely held notion that a high muscle glycogen content prior to a distance run can enhance performance and delay exhaustion. Indeed this has led to the popular belief that "glycogen loading" diets several days prior to a distance run may prolong endurance and performance (see ref 7). Too elevate muscle glycogen, its level is first depleted by running at a moderate to high intensity for a prolonged time. For the next 2-4 days prior to a distance run, a diet high in carbohydrate (pasta and breads) is consumed. During this time daily training bouts can continue. This regimen successfully leads to muscle glyocgen contents higher than normal a phenomenon termed "supercompensation". As can be seen in Table VI (Group 1), human subjects undergoing a "glycogen loading" regimen prior to a distance run of moderate intensity had a high glycogen content and could run significantly longer than subjects consuming a mixed or a low carbohydrate diet. On the other hand, several studies have suggested that diets low in carbohydrates that reduce muscle glycogen may not be at all deleterious or reduce duration of exercise. In one study by Phinney et al. (21), obese individuals were placed on a weight reducing diet consisting of a high quality protein ("protein sparing modified fast"). As shown

**Table V. Effects of Training on Mitochondrial Enzyme
Activity of Rat Skeletal Muscle**

		Fiber types		
Enzyme	Group	IIB	IIA	I
Citrate synthase	Sedentary	10.3	36	23
	Trained	18.5	70	41
Carnitine palmityl-	Sedentary	0.11	0.72	0.63
transferase	Trained	0.20	1.20	1.20
3-hydroxybutyrate	Sedentary	not detectable	0.14	0.34
dehydrogenase	Trained	0.03	0.80	0.88
Cytochrome oxidase	Sedentary	167	830	621
	Trained	339	2041	1347

Enzyme activites in umole/g·min. except cytochrome oxidase which is
in ul O_2/g x min.   Data from Baldwin et al. (16).

**Table VI. Effect of Diet on Muscle Glycogen Content
and Duration of Exercise**

Subjects	Diet	Muscle glycogen content before exercise (umol/g)	Duration of exercise (minutes)
Humans	Normal mixed diet	97	116
	Low carbohydrate diet for 3 days	36	57
	High carbohydrate diet for 3 days (glycogen loading)	103	166
Humans	Normal mixed diet	85	168
	Low carbohydrate diet for 6 weeks	58	249
Rats	Normal chow diet	54	36
	Low carbohydrate diet for 5 weeks	40	47

Data in group 1 from Bergstrom et al. (38), Group 2 from Phinney et
al. (21), and Group 3 from Miller et al. (22).

in Table VI (Group 2), after 6 weeks on this diet muscle glycogen was reduced but the ability of these individuals to remain active at a low intensity exercise increased by 50%. In another study (22), rats fed a low carbohydrate (high fat) diet for 5 weeks were able to tolerate an intense treadmill run longer than rats on a normal diet (Table VI, Group 3). Thus, diets that may actually lower muscle glycogen content are not always associated with reduced performance. It is conceivable that in groups 2 and 3 the primary fuel for the working muscles were provided by free fatty acids and triglycerides resulting in sparing of glycogen. If such was the case, it may help explain why exercise duration was prolonged. It would also re-emphasize that protection of glycogen stores are improtant in delaying the onset of exhaustion during exercise.

More acute dietary manipulations have also been shown to modify exercise performance. When free fatty acid levels were artificially raised in rats by giving corn oil plus heparin, they were able to run about 50% longer than control rats before becoming exhausted (9,23,24). This was associated with a glycogen-sparing effect during the run in that both blood glucose and muscle glycogen declined more slowly. In this association the glycogen-sparing effect was postulated to be due to an enhanced oxidation of fatty acids. On the other hand, glucose ingestion during prolonged light-intensity exercise resulted in augmented uptake and oxidation of glucose by working muscles in association with diminished lipolysis (25,26). It is also thought that exogenous glucose may reduce endogenous glycogen breakdown (26).

Biochemical Regulation of Fuel Utilization during Exercise

The previous sections have indicated that both carbohydrates and lipids can be utilized by muscle during aerobic performance. Due to the small reserve of carbohydrate in the body (Table I), its use as a fuel is limited. To obtain maximal performance during endurance running (i.e., marathon), both carbohydrate and lipid fuels must be used simultaneously (7). As much fatty acid as possible must be oxidized to allow the limited carbohydrate reserves to last for the duration of exercise. Hypoglycemia must be prevented and glucose must be supplied to the brain at all times. This carbohydrate sparing at the expense of fatty acid oxidation has been proposed to be facilitated by a specific intracellular control mechanism. It is well documented that glucose uptake, glycolysis, glycogen breakdown and pyruvate oxidation are inhibited in the heart by oxidation of fatty acids (27). Randle and coworkers (27) proposed that this inhibition of carbohydrate utilization by fatty acids was a general phenomenon. This inhibition is mediated by the rise in muscle acetyl-CoA, citrate and glucose-6-phosphate during fatty acid oxidation (Figure 5). An increase in the acetyl-CoA ratio will inhibit pyruvate dehydrogenase and reduce carbohydrate oxidation; citrate produced within the mitochondria will be transported into the cytoplasm and will inhibit phosphofructokinase thereby restricting glycolysis; and the resultant rise in glucose-6-phosphate can inhibit hexokinase restricting glucose uptake by

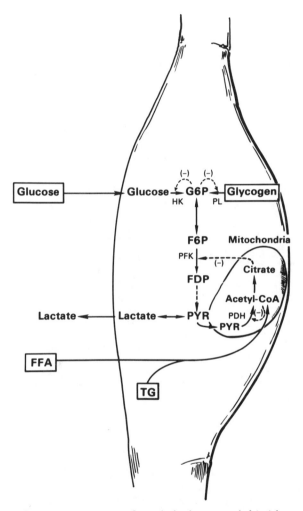

Figure 5 - Interaction of carbohydrate snd lipid metabolism during exercise. G6P, glucose--6-phosphate;F6P, fructose-6--phosphate; FDP, fructose-1,6-diphosphate; Pyr, Pyruvate; FFA, free fatty acid TG, triglyceride; HK, hexokinase; PL, phosphorylase; PFK, phosphofructokinase and PDH, pyruvate dehydrogenase.

muscle. There is also evidence that a rise in glucose-6-phosphate may inhibit glycogen breakdown (7). Although this mechanism is operative in cardiac muscle, studies using skeletal muscle (incubated in vitro or perfused in situ) have not always demonstrated an inhibitory effect of fatty acids (or other lipid fuels) on glucose metabolism (28-30). When demonstrated, it has been confined to those muscles that have a high capacity to oxidize lipid fuels such as type I and IIA fibers (29,30).

As noted previously, like skeletal muscle, glycogen depletion in liver during endurance exercise is much less in trained animals and in animals who have had free fatty acids artificially elevated. No evidence exists that the mechanism proposed by Randle to account for the inhibition of carbohydrate metabolism in muscle by oxidation of fatty acids is operative in the liver. Thus other factors must be responsible for the slower rate of liver glycogen depletion in these situations. Such factors may include a smaller increase in catecholamine levels, a smaller reduction in insulin levels, and a smaller reduction in blood flow to the liver during exercise (19,20).

Carbohydrate Metabolism Following Exercise

Following exercise, glucose uptake by the previously working muscles does not fall to pre-exercise levels but remains elevated (31). Teleologically, this would ensure that muscle glycogen stores depleted during exercise are rapidly replenished upon cessation of exercise. Recent studies in the rat have shown that following exercise, glucose transport and glycogen synthesis in skeletal muscle are enhanced due at least, in part, to an increase in insulin sensitivity (32-36). It was also shown that the increase in insulin sensitivity occurs predominantly in muscle fibers that are deglycogenated during exercise, in other words, in the active muscles (33). The precise mechanism for the increase in insulin sensitivity following exercise is not known nor is it associated with an increase in insulin binding to its receptor on the muscle cell (34-36).

Summary

During the early minutes of exercise, carbohydrate (plasma glucose and muscle glycogen) is the predominant fuel for the working muscles. When the exercise is prolonged and intensive, carbohydrate remains a predominant fuel with lipids (plasma free fatty acids and muscle triglycerides) being of lesser importance. When the exercise is of moderate intensity, lipids eventually become the primary fuel as carbohydrate stores are reduced.

After training, which increases the oxidative capacity of the muscles, lipid fuels become the major energy source of the working muscles during prolonged exertion sparing carbohydrate utilization.

Both low and high carbonydrate diets can increase exercise duration; however, low carbohydrate diets may diminish the power output or VO_2 max during exertion. Althouth diets high in carbohydrate or fat (low carbohydrate) may enhance exercise performance, it is recommended that a mixed diet be consumed by those undertaking exercise for health benefits or weight reduction.

During recovery from exercise, glucose uptake by the previously working muscles remains elevated. This is due, in part, to an increase in the sensitivity of muscle to insulin, facilitating glycogen repletion.

Literature Cited

1. Ruderman, N.B. & Haudenschild, C. (1984) Diabetes as an atherogenic factor. Progress in Cardiovascular Diseases 26:373-412.
2. Richter, E.A., Ruderman, N.B. and Schneider, S.H. (1984) Diabetes and Exercise. Am. J. Med. 70:201-209.
3. Gollnick, P.D. (1977) Free fatty acid turnover and the quantability of substrates as a limiting factor in prolonged exercise. Ann. N.Y. Acad. Sci. 301:64-71.
4. Goodman, M.N. and Ruderman, N.B. (1982) Influence of muscle use on amino acid metabolism. In, Exercise and Sport Science Reviews, ed. by R.L. Terjung, The Franklin Institute, Philadelphia, PA, 1-26.
5. Cahill, G.F. (1970) Starvation in man. New Eng. J. Med. 282:668-675, 6. Owen, O.E. and Reichard, G.A. (1971) Human forearm metabolism during progressive starvation. J. Clin, Invest. 50:1536-1545.
7. Newsholme, E.A., and Leech, A.R. (1983) Metabolism in Exercise. In, Biochemistry for the Medical Sciences John Wiley and sons, New York, Chapter 9.
8. Newsholme, E.A. (1977) The regulation of intracellular and extracellular fuel supply during sustained exercise. Ann. N.Y. Acad. Sci. 301:81-91, 9. Holloszy, J.O., Rennie, M.J., Hickson, R.C., Conlee, R.K. and Hagberg, J.M. (1977) Consequences of the biochemical adaptations to endurance exercise. Ann. N.Y. Acad. Sci. 301:440-450.
10. Saltin, B., Henriksson, J., Nygaard, E. and Andersen, P. (1977) Fiber types and metabolic potentials of skeletal muscles in sedentary man and endurance runners. Ann. N.Y. Acad. Sci. 301:3-29.
11. Felig, P. and Wahren, J. (1975) Fuel homeostasis in exercise. N. Engl. J. Med. 293:1078-1084.
12. Wahren, J.: Glucose turnover during exercise in man (1977) Ann. N.Y. Acad. Sci. 301:45-53.
13. Wahren, J., Felig, P. and Hagenfeldt, L. (1978) Physical exercise and fuel homeostasis in diabetes mellitus. Diabetologia, 14:213-222.
14. Berger, M., Hagg, S. and Ruderman, N.B. (1975) Glucose metabolism in perfused skeletal muscle. Biochem. J. 146:231-238.
15. Essen, B. (1977) Intramuscular substrate utilization during prolonged exercise. Ann. N.Y. Acad. Sci. 301:30-44.
16. Baldwin, K.M., Klinkerfuss, G.H., Terjung, R.L., Mole, P.A. and Holloszy, J.O. (1972) Respiratory capacity of white, red, and intermediate muscle: adaptive response to exercise. Am. J. Physiol. 222:373-378.

17. Holloszy, J.O. and Coyle, E.F. (1984) Adaptations of
     skeletal muscle to endurance exercise and their metabolic
     consequences. J. Appl. Physiol. 56:831-838.
18. Baldwin, K.M., Winder, W.W., Terjung, R.L., and Holloszy,
     J.O. (1973) Glycolytic enzymes in different types of
     skeletal muscle: adaptation to exercise. Am. J. Physiol.
     225:962-966.
19. Koivisto, V., R. Hendler, R., Nadel, E. & Felig, P. (1982)
     Influence of physical training on the fuel-hormone response
     to prolonged low intensity exercise. Metabolism 31;192-197.
20. Baldwin, K.M. Fitts, R.H., Booth, F.W., Winder, W.W. &
     Holloszy, J.O. (1975) Depletion of muscle and liver
     glycogen during exercise. Pflugers Arch.354;203-212 1975.
21. Phinney, S.D., Harton, E.S., Sims, E.A., Hanson, J.S.,
     Danforth, E. & La Grange, B.M. (1984) Capacity for moderate
     exercise in obese subjects after adaptation to a
     hpyocaloric, ketogenic diet. J. Clin. Investigation
     66;1152-1161.
22. Miller, W.C., Bryce, R.K. & Conlee, R.K. (1984) Adaptations
     to a hight-fat diet that increases exercise endurance in
     male rats. J. Appl. Physiol. 56; 78-83.
23. Hickson, R.C., Rennie, M.J., Conlee, R.K., Winder, W.W. &
     Holloszy, J.O. (1977) Effects of increased plasma fatty
     acids on glycogen utilization and endurance. J. Appl.
     Physiol. 43, 829-833.
24. Rennie, M.J., Winder, W.W. & Holloszy, J.O. (1976) A
     sparing effect of increased plasma fatty acids on muscle and
     liver glycogen content in exercising rat. Biochem. J. 156:
     647-655.
25. Ahlborg, G. & Felig, P. (1976) Influence of glucose
     ingestion on fuel-hormone response during prolonged
     exercise. J. App;. Physiol. 41: 683-688.
26. Krezentowski, G., Freddy, P., Luyckx, A.S., Lacroix, M.
     Mosora, F. & Lefebvre, P.J. (1984) Effects of physical
     training on utilization of a glucose load given orally
     during exercise. Am, J. Physiol. 246, E412-E417.
27. Randle, P.J., Garland, P.B., Hales, C.N., Newsholme, E.A.,
     Denton, R.M. &   Pogson, C.I. (1966) Interactions of
     metabolism and physiological role of insulin.Rec. Prog.
     Horm. Res. 22, 1-44.
28. Goodman, M.N., Berger, M. & Ruderman, N.B. (1974) Glucose
     metabolism in rat skeletal muscle at rest. Diabetes 23;
     881-888.
29. Maizels, E.Z., Ruderman, N.B., Goodman, M.N. & Lau, D.
     (1977) Effects of acetoacetate on glucose metabolism in
     soleus and extensor digitorum longus muscles of the rat.
     Biochem, J. 162; 557-568.
30. Rennie, M.J. & Holloszy, J.O. (1977) Inhibition of glucose
     uptake and glycogenolysis by availability of oleate in well-
     oxygenated perfused skeletal muscle. Biochem. J. 168;
     161-170.
31. Wahren, J., Felig, P., Hendler, R. & Ahlborg, G. (1973)
     Glucose and amino acid metabolism during recovery after
     exercise. J. Appl. Physiol. 34; 838-845.

32. Ivy, J. & Holloszy, J.O. (1981) Persistent increase in glucose uptake by rat skeletal muscle following exercise. Am. J. Physiol. 241, C200-C203.

33. Richter, E.A., Garetto, L.P., Goodman, M.N. & Ruderman, N.B. (1982) Muscle glucose metabolism following exercise in the rat. J. Clin. Investigation. 69, 785-793.

34. Garetto, L.P., Richter, E.A., Goodman, M.N. & Ruderman, N.B. (1983) Enhanced insullin sensitivity of skeletal muscle following exercise. In: Biochemistry of Exercise, ed. by H. Knuttgen, J. Vogel and J. Poortman. Champaign, IL., p. 681-687.

35. Horton, E.G. (1983) Increased insulin sensitivity without altered insulin binding in rat soleus muscle. Excerpta Med. Int. Cong. Ser. 577, 182.

36. Tan, M. & Bonen, A. (1983) Exercise enhances glycogenesis in muscle without affecting their insulin binding and 2-deoxyglucose uptake. Excerpta Med. Int. Ser. 5577, 182.

37. Newsholme, E.A. (1983) Control of metabolism and integration of fuel supply for the marathon runner. In: Biochemistry of Exercise, ed. by H. Knuttgen, J. Vogel and J. Poortman. Champaign, IL., p.144-150.

38. Bergstrom, J., Hermansen, L. & Hultman, E. (1967) Diet, muscle glycogen and physical performance. Acta. Physiol. Scand. 71, 140-150.

RECEIVED May 14, 1985

Protein and Amino Acid Metabolism During Exercise

Donald K. Layman and Melissa K. Hendrix

Department of Foods and Nutrition, Division of Nutritional Sciences, University of Illinois, Urbana, IL 61801

Athletes associate performance with diet. Meat became a staple of ancient Greek and Roman athletes as they attempted to achieve the strength and endurance of carnivorous members of the animal kingdom. As knowledge of nutrition and muscle physiology increased, athletes became convinced that to increase muscle mass and strength required increased dietary protein. However, nutrition textbooks (1,2) and the Recommended Dietary Allowances (RDA's) established by the National Academy of Sciences (3) state that there is little or no need for extra protein for exercise.

Review of the nutrition and exercise literature indicates that physical activity produces changes in protein metabolism. A few of these changes are increased urinary nitrogen, increased nitrogen in sweat, and increased protein mass of muscles. These physiological changes, which suggest an increased need for dietary protein, together with the renewed popular interest in exercise have led to a reevaluation of protein utilization during exercise. Aspects of this topic have been addressed in other recent reviews (4,5,6).

To examine the influence of exercise on protein metabolism, it is important to consider the differences between types of exercise. The previous chapters by Terjung and Goodman have examined the effects of exercise intensity and duration on different muscles and the primary fuels required for specific activities. For the purpose of this chapter, exercise will be classified as anaerobic or aerobic. These terms indicate metabolic differences and imply differences in intensity and duration. Anaerobic activities are of brief duration and at, or approaching, maximum exertion. Anaerobic training emphasizes strength and frequently results in muscle hypertrophy. Aerobic exercise features prolonged activities at less than maximum exertion. Training emphasizes endurance work and results in increased oxidative capacity of the muscles with little or no change in muscle mass. Thus, the type of exercise can influence muscle mass and the amount of muscle proteins and presumably the needs for dietary protein.

To conceptualize amino acid metabolism, it is useful to consider a model which describes the flux of amino acids through

0097-6156/86/0294-0045$06.00/0

free amino acid pools. The most commonly used model is one that
features a single amino acid pool which accounts for the flux of
amino acids to protein synthesis or oxidation from a single
homogeneous pool (7,8).

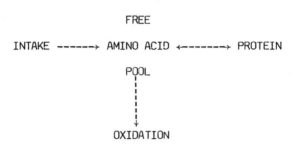

As the model suggests, the dietary need for amino acids is
determined by the rates of depletion of the free amino acid pool
by oxidation or synthesis of protein. During steady state
conditions, the contribution to the free pool from dietary intake
and protein breakdown should be exactly balanced by the flux out
of the pool to synthesis and oxidation. Any condition that
increases deposition of protein in the body or the rate of amino
acid oxidation should produce an increased need for protein. For
example, muscle hypertrophy is dependent on a positive balance of
the protein turnover process. If synthesis of protein exceeds the
catabolism of protein, then muscle mass will increase and the free
amino acid pool would be depleted. Thus, a net increase in
protein requires an increase in intake or a decrease in oxidation.
Likewise, the same arguments hold for an increase in oxidation of
amino acids.

Amino Acid Metabolism Associated with Anaerobic Exercise

Specific exercise such as weightlifting can increase muscle mass
(9,10). While the potential to develop muscle mass is
established, the metabolic changes that lead to these changes
remain unclear. Relatively few studies have examined amino acid
metabolism during exercise-induced hypertrophy. The primary
reason for the lack of information is the absence of a convenient
animal model for weightlifting studies. Human studies utilizing
nonradioactive, stable isotopes have not yet been done.
    While few studies exist that are designed to evaluate amino
acid metabolism during and after anaerobic exercise, some insight
into changes in protein synthesis can be gained from studies that
produce muscle hypertrophy using novel surgical procedures or
mechanical stimulations. One series of studies from the
laboratory of A.L. Goldberg examined hypertrophy of specific
muscles after surgical removal of a synergistic muscle (11,12).
These investigators utilized the triad of muscles extending from
the knee to the ankle on the back of the hind limb of rats. These
three muscles, the soleus, plantaris, and gastrocnemius, serve to
extend the ankle joint. Specifically, Goldberg and his colleagues

severed the achilles tendon of the gastrocnemius and observed the changes in protein synthesis in the soleus and plantaris muscles as these muscles hypertrophied under the functional overload in an attempt to maintain the ability of the animal to extend the foot. This treatment produced a 40% increase in the weight of the soleus and a 25% increase in the weight of the plantaris by 5 days after they were surgically overloaded. These investigators demonstrated that there was a corresponding increase in protein content and related increases in RNA content, ribosome activity, and incorporation of amino acids into protein. They concluded that muscle hypertrophy was produced by a dramatic increase in protein synthesis.

A second experimental model that may approximate weightlifting exercise is "stretch-induced hypertrophy" (13,14). As the term implies, stretch-induced hypertrophy consists of producing muscle hypertrophy by forcing a muscle into full extension through the use of weights or a plaster cast. The metabolic changes are similar to the surgical model. Stretch will produce a rapid increase in muscle weight and protein content and in the rate of protein synthesis (Table 1). These investigators estimated the rate of protein degradation and concluded that protein degradation was also elevated but hypertrophy occurred because the increase in synthesis exceeded the increase in degradation (14).

Table 1. Changes in Protein Turnover in Anterior Latissimus Dorsi Muscles of Chickens During Stretch-Induced Hypertrophy

Time	Synthesis	Degradation
(days)	(%/day)	
0	16.5	16.5
1	33.0	21.6
3	32.5	23.0
7	31.3	27.5

Synthesis measured using the constant infusion of ^{14}C-proline and degradation calculated as the difference between the rate of synthesis and the rate of protein accretion. From Laurent et al. (14).

These experimental models indicate that muscle hypertrophy occurs through increases in protein synthesis and suggest that weightlifting should require increased dietary protein. The confusion is derived from the interpretation of the quantity of protein needed to meet this increased need. The RDA's state that "there is little evidence that muscular activity increases the need for protein, except by the small amount required for the development of muscles during conditioning." The amount has been

reported to be a maximum of 7 grams of additional protein per day
(15).

The impact of 7 grams of protein per day on the American diet
is virtually negligible. The daily protein needs range from
approximately 40 to 90 grams per day (0.8 grams per kilogram body
weight), while the average American consumes nearly twice the need
or about 110 grams per day. Thus, the increased need for muscle
hypertrophy should be adequately met by normal intakes without
supplementation.

Though the amount of muscle protein gained per day during
weight training does not justify an increased protein intake, many
athletes believe that high levels of protein are essential to
stimulate maximum muscle development. However, as shown in
Fig. 1, intakes of protein above the requirement produce no
stimulation of protein synthesis. By feeding different levels of
protein to rodents, we found that maximum muscle mass and the
maximum rate of protein synthesis were achieved at relatively low
levels of dietary protein and intakes two or three times this
level produced no additional stimulation (16).

Goldberg and his colleagues provided further evidence that
dietary protein is not a limiting factor for muscle hypertrophy
(12). Using their surgical model for compensatory hypertrophy,
they found that the increase in protein synthesis and muscle mass
could occur during periods of total starvation. Thus, hypertrophy
of specific muscles was produced by the selective training,
workload, or stretch put on that muscle and was not dependent on
diet. Obviously, the total muscle mass of the body cannot be
increased during total starvation, but Goldberg's work suggests
that the body is capable of redistributing protein to achieve a
functional need of specific muscles.

In summary, anaerobic exercise can induce muscle hypertrophy
which requires some additional protein beyond maintenance needs.
However, the rate of protein accretion suggests that the increased
need is not more than 7 grams of protein per day. Relatively few
studies have determined changes in protein turnover during and
after anaerobic exercise. It has not been established if any
changes occur in the efficiency of protein gain during anaerobic
exercise or if the timing of protein intake relative to the
exercise is important.

Amino Acid Metabolism Associated with Aerobic Training

The role of protein and amino acids as a source of energy during
exercise is unclear. Astrand (17) suggested that "fuels for
working muscles are limited to carbohydrate and fat." Statements
such as this one suggest that protein is not used as a fuel.
However, if we examine the composition of the American diet for
nongrowing adults this statement appears to be an
oversimplification. Protein accounts for approximately 12% of the
daily caloric intake with 46% derived from carbohydrates and 42%
from lipids (2). The potential for use of amino acids for energy
was further supported by Cahill (18). In his publication
"Starvation in Man," he reported amino acids to be an important
energy source during starvation. Specifically, protein breakdown
in skeletal muscle served as an important source of substrate for
the process of gluconeogenesis.

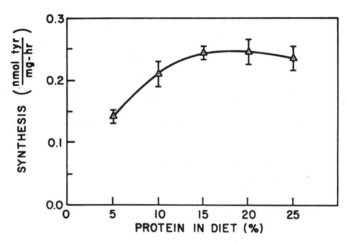

Figure 1. The rate of protein synthesis in soleus muscles from rats fed different levels of dietary protein. Synthesis was measured as the incorporation of a radioactive amino acid (tyrosine) into muscle proteins. Data from Ref. 16.

Reviews by Ruderman (19) and Adibi (20,21) indicate that the branched-chain amino acids, particularly leucine, have an important role along with alanine in gluconeogenesis. Leucine and the other two branched-chain amino acids are catabolized in skeletal muscle. The nitrogen that is removed from the branched-chain amino acids in skeletal muscle is combined with pyruvate and returned to the liver as alanine. In the liver the nitrogen is removed for urea production and the carbon chain is utilized as substrate for synthesis of glucose. Adibi et al. (22) reported that during the catabolic conditions of starvation, oxidation of leucine and fatty acids increases in skeletal muscles. While glucose oxidation is reduced, the capacity for oxidation of the fatty acid palmitate more than doubled, and leucine oxidation increased by a factor of six.

Ahlborg et al. (23) extended these findings using six untrained adult males exercised at 30% VO_{2max} on a bicycle ergometer. They examined changes in blood levels of amino acids before and after 40 minutes of aerobic exercise (Table 2). They measured arterial/venous differences across the leg muscles versus the splanchnic bed and found significant differences in blood levels of alanine and the branched-chain amino acids. Alanine is removed from the blood by the liver for gluconeogenesis and the uptake was increased by exercise. On the other hand, leucine and isoleucine are released by the liver and taken up by skeletal muscles. Both the release by liver and the uptake by muscles are increased during exercise. These data demonstrate a change in amino acid flux during exercise which is an increase in the release of branched-chain amino acids from viseral tissues to skeletal muscles and the return of alanine as a precursor for glucose synthesis.

Table 2. Arterial-Venous Difference in Amino Acid Uptake During Exercise

Amino Acid	Splanchnic Exchange (umol/min)		Leg Exchange (umol/min)	
	Rest	40 min.	Rest	40 min.
Alanine	58	90	-30	-45
Leucine	- 2.2	- 8.8	- 0.8	13.2
Isoleucine	- 1.0	- 2.9	- 0.4	8.2

Six untrained males were exercised for 4 hours at 30% VO_{2max} on a bicycle ergometer. Positive numbers indicate uptake and negative numbers indicate release. From Ahlborg et al. (24).

Subsequently, Dohm et al. (24) demonstrated an increased production of carbon dioxide from leucine during exercise. They found a 50% increase in CO_2 production in muscle tissue from trained rats. The study by Dohm et al. (24) utilized a motor-driven treadmill with an eight degree incline and ran the animals at 35 meters per minute for 60 minutes per day, 6 days per week. These experimental conditions produce an exercise intensity of 75-80% of VO_{2max}. This program was used for 6 to 8 weeks.

The effects of exercise on branched-chain amino acids may be unique. The branched-chain amino acids are essential in the diet and are uniquely catabolized in skeletal muscles. These amino acids may provide an energy source for muscles or may serve an intermediate role in maintaining blood glucose through production of alanine via transamination with pyruvate in muscles (19).

The uniqueness of leucine can be further demonstrated by examining muscle protein synthesis. We have shown that leucine has the ability to stimulate protein synthesis in muscles during catabolic conditions such as starvation (25). Using a large dose of leucine, protein synthesis can be stimulated 50% in muscles from starved rats. The significance of this effect remains controversial; however, the in vitro activity is clear and emphasizes the unique metabolic potential of leucine.

These studies have demonstrated that exercise affects amino acid metabolism with specific effects on leucine. Dohm et al. (26) extended these findings by studying the influence of exercise on protein synthesis in perfused rat muscles. They demonstrated that exercise decreased the rate of protein synthesis and that the level of exertion was important to the magnitude of the effect. Mild exercise produced by swimming rats for one hour decreased protein synthesis by 17%. While more intense treadmill running reduced synthesis by 30% and an exhaustive run of three hours inhibited synthesis by 70%. These data suggest that exercise may produce a catabolic condition in muscles which would make amino acids available for oxidation and that this effect is dependent on the intensity and duration of the exercise.

Using exhaustive running, Dohm et al. (27) examined the magnitude of the catabolic effect. They ran rats at 28 meters per minute for 4 hours and measured the excretion of urinary urea and 3-methylhistidine (Table 3). Urea excretion increased by 31% during the first 12 hours after the exhaustive bout of exercise, but returned to normal during the next 12 hours. It is interesting to note the delayed effect. During exercise there is decreased renal clearance and the blood urea increases. Post-exercise urea increases in the urine. Urinary 3-methylhistidine, which is an indicator of the rate of muscle protein breakdown, also increased after the exercise. However, the increase in the 3-methylhistidine did not occur until 12 to 36 hours after the exercise. Based on these findings, these investigators estimated that 15 to 20% of the energy for endurance exercise may come from protein. If this is true aerobic exercise could double the dietary need for protein.

The suggestion that exercise produces a catabolic condition was further supported by Rennie et al. (28) studying aerobic exercise in humans. They exercised six male subjects on a treadmill for 3 3/4 hours at 50% VO_{2max} and measured the rates

Table 3. Effect of Exhaustive Running on Protein Metabolism in
          Rats

Time After Exercise	Urea Excretion (mmol/kg)		3-Methylhistidine Excretion (mmol/kg)	
	Control	Exercised	Control	Exercised
First 12 hrs.	10.0	13.1*	9.4	10.4
Second 12 hrs.	15.8	17.7	7.8	11.4*
Second 24 hrs.	24.6	28.4	17.8	21.4*

From Dohm et al. (27).

of protein synthesis and degradation (Table 4). During the
exercise, the rate of synthesis decreased by 14% while the rate of
degradation increased by 54%. This study is also important
because it is one of the few studies to make measurements both
during and after the exercise bout. Post-exercise the rate of
synthesis increased above the initial levels suggesting the
recovery pattern after the exercise. These post-exercise results
are important in assessing the impact of exercise on the
nutritional requirement.

Table 4. Protein Turnover at Rest, During, and After Exercise

	Synthesis	Degradation
	(mg of nitrogen/kg x hr)	
Rest	33.0 + 2.0	26.5 + 2.1
Exercised	28.4 + 1.6	40.9 + 2.6
Post-exercise	40.3 + 1.9	35.4 + 1.2

Six male subjects were exercised on a treadmill for 3.75 hours
at 50% VO_{2max}. From Rennie et al. (28).

     The mechanism that produces increased amino acid oxidation
during exercise is unknown. White and Brooks (29) demonstrated
a relationship of amino acid oxidation to use of blood glucose.
Concomitant with increases in the intensity of exercise and
leucine oxidation, the oxidation of glucose and alanine increased.
These data in combination with the earlier reports of increased
flux of leucine to skeletal muscles and alanine from muscles to
the liver suggest that the oxidation of amino acids may be linked
to the need for glucose and to generation of substrates for
gluconeogenesis.

The relationship of amino acid oxidation to carbohydrate status was examined by Lemon and Mullin (30). Employing six physically active men, these investigators manipulated the dietary intake of carbohydrate to determine the effects of aerobic exercise on protein catabolism. Their diets consisted of a single carbohydrate-free meal followed by an overnight fast or three days of high carbohydrate feeding. Based on previously published reports, these diets were assumed to produce, respectively, depletion or elevation of muscle glycogen stores. They estimated protein catabolism from serum urea concentration and the nitrogen content of sweat before and after 1 hour of moderate intensity bicycle exercise. The exercise bout produced no change in serum urea in the group fed the high carbohydrate diet, but did produce some loss of urea by sweat (Table 5). However, under the same exercise conditions following the carbohydrate-free meal, these men experienced significant elevations in both blood urea and sweat nitrogen. These data further suggest that the catabolism of amino acids during exercise is associated with changes in glucose availability.

Table 5. Loss of Nitrogen Via Sweat after Aerobic Exercise

	Sweat Urea (mg nitrogen/hr)
Rest	10
CHO-Loaded	600
CHO-Depleted	1450

Six males were exercised on a bicycle ergometer at 61% VO_{2max} for 1 hour. From Lemon & Mullin (30).

Protein Requirements for Endurance Exercise

The impact of aerobic exercise on protein requirements remains uncertain. Exercise clearly can disrupt protein metabolism, both protein turnover and amino acid oxidation. However, it remains to be determined if these effects are acute effects of exhaustive exercise or if moderate exercise in trained individuals still produces increased oxidation of amino acids.

The work by Wolfe et al. (31,32) serves to emphasize some of these problems. They utilized a mild bicycle exercise and examined the effects on leucine oxidation and urea production. Four untrained men were exercised for 105 minutes on a bicycle ergometer at an intensity designed to maintain a heart rate of 110 beats/minute (approximately 30% VO_{2max}). Comparing a pre-exercise rest period to immediately post-exercise, they found a 2- to 3-fold increase in the production of CO_2 from leucine, but they found no increase in urea production. They also determined that while mild exercise increased oxidation of leucine, there was no effect on the catabolism of another essential amino acid, lysine (32). These studies demonstrate that the effect of exercise on leucine oxidation can occur at very low exercise intensity, but they also suggest that exercise may have a unique effect on leucine metabolism, at least under mild exercise conditions.

A recent paper further questions the potential impact of exercise on protein requirement (33). These investigators state that while pertrubations in protein and amino acid metabolism may exist during the initial adaptation to exercise, no one has demonstrated a long-term catabolic effect of exercise on lean body mass. Further, they suggest that the results from many of the exercise studies are confounded by a failure to define or control energy intake. In their experiments using low intensity exercise, they found a negative nitrogen balance in young men receiving a marginal protein intake (0.57 g/kg). Using the same protein intake and exercise levels, nitrogen balance became positive when the energy intake was increased by 15%. This effect was moderated by additional exercise. These researchers concluded that the major effect of exercise on nitrogen balance is a transient change during the initial adaptation to a new exercise program but that with adequate energy intake the efficiency of protein utilization actually improves during exercise.

Preliminary work in our laboratory suggests that the effect of exercise on leucine oxidation is not just a transient effect of beginning an exercise program, and that the magnitude of the effect is dependent on the duration of the exercise (Fig. 2). Male rats were trained to run on a treadmill at 28 meters/minute (approximately 80% VO_{2max}) for 50 or 120 minutes/day. After 6 weeks of training the rate of leucine oxidation was determined. The curves in Figure 2 indicate that exercise increases leucine oxidation and that the stimulation may be directly related to duration of exercise.

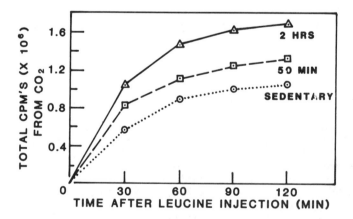

Figure 2. The effects of the duration of exercise on the production of radioactive CO_2 from ^{14}C-labeled leucine (see text).

Summary

Early research on protein requirements established that protein
was not a major fuel for exercise, and that fat and carbohydrates
were quantitatively more important. The Recommended Dietary
Allowance (RDA) for protein is 0.8 grams per kilogram of body
weight (0.36 grams/pound). These guidelines suggest that protein
needs range from approximately 40 to 90 grams per day depending on
body weight. Currently, the average daily intake of protein in
the United States is 100-110 grams per day, which suggests that
supplemental protein is unlikely to be necessary for routine
exercise. However, recent experiments with exhaustive exercise
have raised additional questions about the needs for protein
during aerobic exercise.

Exercise is known to have acute catabolic effects on muscle
protein turnover. During exercise protein snythesis is depressed
which leads to protein catabolism. However, the impact of a
relatively short exercise bout on 24-hour protein needs is unclear.
Anaerobic exercise can produce hypertrophy of specific muscles
depending on the type of training utilized. The hypertrophy is
due to a positive balance in protein turnover which appears to be
produced by an increase in the rate of protein synthesis after
exercise. The increased need for protein during anaerobic
exercise is unlikely to be more than 7 grams per day.

Aerobic exercise usually increases the percentage of muscle
mass due to a decrease in body fat, but produces no absolute
change in the amount of muscle. Aerobic exercise has been shown
to alter protein metabolism including increases in amino acid
oxidation with specific effects on the branched-chain amino acid
leucine, increased urinary urea, and increased sweat nitrogen.
The magnitude of each of these effects appears to depend on the
intensity and duration of the activity with larger effects
occurring at more exhaustive levels. The absolute effects of
aerobic exercise on the requirements for protein or a specific
essential amino acid remain to be determined. However, because
aerobic exercise produces changes in amino acid metabolism, it is
important for individuals with the highest protein needs, such as
growing children and adolescents, women during pregnancy and
lactation, and individuals on low caloric diets, to maintain
adequate protein intakes when participating in aerobic exercise.

Literature Cited

1. Guthrie, H. (1983) In: Introductory Nutrition. Fifth
    Edition. C.V. Mosby Co., St. Louis, MO.

2. Whitney, E.N. (1982) In: Nutrition Concepts and
    Controversies. Second Edition. West Publishing Co., St.
    Paul, MN.

3. Recommended Dietary Allowances. (1980) Protein and amino
    acids. Ninth Edition. National Academy of Sciences,
    Washington, D.C., pp. 39-54.

4. Lemon, P.W.R. & Nagle, F.J. (1981) Effects of exercise on
    protein and amino acid metabolism. Med. Sci. Sports &
    Exercise 13, 141-149.

5. Goodman, M.N. & Ruderman, N.B. (1982) Influence of muscle
    use on amino acid metabolism. In: Exercise and Sport
    Sciences Reviews. R.L. Terjung, ed., pp. 1-26. The Franklin
    Institute, Philadelphia, PA.

6. Evans, W.J., Fisher, E.C., Hoerr, R.A. & Young, V.R. (1983)
    Protein metabolism and endurance exercise. Physician &
    Sportmedicine 11, 63-72.

7. Waterlow, J.C., Garlick, P.J. & Millward, D.J. (1978) In:
    Protein Turnover in Mammalian Tissues and in the Whole Body.
    Elsevier/North Holland, NY.

8. Wolfe, R.R. (1984) In: Tracers in Metabolic Research.
    Radioisotope and Stable Isotope/Mass Spectrometry Methods.
    Alan R. Liss, Inc., NY.

9. Misner, J.E., Boileau, R.A., Massey, B.H. & Mayhew, J.L.
    (1974) Alterations in the body composition of adult men
    during selected physical training programs. J. Amer.
    Geriatric Soc. 22, 33-38.

10. Goldspink, G. (1964) The combined effects of exercise and
    reduced food intake on skeletal muscle fibers. J. Cell.
    Comp. Physiol. 63, 209-216.

11. Goldberg, A.L. (1967) Work-induced growth of skeletal
    muscle in normal and hypophysectomized rats. Am. J. Physiol.
    213, 1193-1198.

12. Goldberg, A.L. (1971) Biochemical events during hypertrophy
    of skeletal muscle. In: Cardiac Hypertrophy. N.R. Alpert,
    ed., pp. 301-314. Academic Press, NY.

13. Goldspink, D.F. (1978) The influence of passive stretch on
    the growth and protein turnover of the denervated extensor
    digitorium longus muscle. Biochem. J. 174, 595-602.

14. Laurent, G.J., Sparrow, M.P. & Millward, D.J. (1978) Muscle
    protein turnover in the adult fowl II. Changes in rates of
    protein synthesis and breakdown during hypertrophy of the
    anterior and posterior latissimus dorsi muscle. Biochem. J.
    176, 407-417.

15. Durmin, J.V.G.A. (1978) Protein requirements and physical
    activity. In: Nutrition, Physical Fitness, and Health. J.
    Parizkova & V.A. Rogozkin, eds., pp. 53-60. University Park
    Press, Baltimore, MD.

16. Smith, C.K., Durschlag, R.P. & Layman, D.K. (1982) Response of skeletal muscle protein synthesis and breakdown to levels of dietary protein and fat during growth in weanling rats. J. Nutr. 112, 255-262.

17. Astrand, P.O. (1979) Nutrition and physical performance. In: Nutrition and the World Food Problem, p. 63. Basel:Karger Press.

18. Cahill, G.F. (1970) Starvation in man. The New England Journal Medicine, March 19, 668-675.

19. Ruderman, N.B. (1975) Muscle amino acid metabolism and gluconeogenesis. Ann. Rev. Med. 26, 245-258.

20. Adibi, S.A. (1976) Metabolism of branched-chain amino acids in altered nutrition. Metab. 25, 1287-1302.

21. Hogg, S.A., Morse, E.L. & Adibi, S.A. (1982) Effect of exercise on rates of oxidation, turnover, and plasma clearance of leucine in human subjects. Amer. J. Physiol. 242, E407-E410.

22. Adibi, S.A., Krzysik, B.A. & Morse, E.L. (1974) Oxidative energy metabolism in the skeletal muscle: biochemical and ultrastructural evidence for adaptive changes. J. Lab. Clin. Invest. 83, 548-562.

23. Ahlborg, G., Felig, P., Hagenfeldt, L., Hendler, R. & Wahren, J. (1974) Substrate turnover during prolonged exercise in man. J. Clin. Invest. 53, 1080-1090.

24. Dohm, G.L., Hecker, A.L., Brown, W.E., Klain, G.J., Puente, F.R., Askew, E.W. & Beecher, G.R. (1977) Adaptation of protein metabolism to endurance training. Biochem. J. 164, 705-708.

25. Hong, S.C. & Layman, D.K. (1984) Effects of leucine on in vitro protein synthesis and degradation in rat skeletal muscles. J. Nutr. 114, 1204-1212.

26. Dohm, G.L., Tapscott, E.B., Barakat, H.A. & Kasperek, G.J. (1982) Measurement of in vivo protein synthesis in rats during an exercise bout. Biochem. Med. 27, 367-373.

27. Dohm, G.L., Williams, R.T., Kasperek, G.J. & van Rij, A.M. (1982) Increased excretion of urea and N^τ-methylhistidine by rats and humans after a bout of exercise. J. Appl. Physiol. 52, 27-33.

28. Rennie, M.J., Edwards, R.N.T., Krywawych, S., Davies, C.T.M., Halliday, D., Waterlow, J.C. & Millward, D.J. (1981) Effect of exercise on protein turnover in man. Clin. Sci. 61, 627-639.

29.   White, T.P. & Brooks, G.A. (1981) U^{14}-C glucose,
      -alanine, and -leucine oxidation in rats at rest and two
      intensities of running. Am. J. Physiol. 240, E155-E165.

30.   Lemon, P.W.R. & Mullin, J.P. (1980) Effect of initial
      muscle glycogen levels on protein catabolism during
      exercise. J. Appl. Physiol. 48, 624-629.

31.   Wolfe, R.R., Goodenough, R.D., Wolfe, M.H., Royle, G.T. &
      Nadel, E.R. (1982) Isotopic analysis of leucine and urea
      metabolism in exercising humans. J. Appl. Physiol. 52,
      458-466.

32.   Wolfe, R.R., Wolfe, M.H., Nadel, E.R. & Shaw, J.H.F. (1984)
      Isotopic determination of amino acid-urea interactions in
      exercise in humans. J. Appl. Physiol. 56, 221-229.

33.   Butterfield, G.E. & Calloway, D.H. (1984) Physical activity
      improves protein utilization in young men. Brit. J. Nutr.
      51, 171-184.

RECEIVED June 21, 1985

The Effect of Exercise on Lipid and Lipoprotein Metabolism

P. M. Kris-Etherton

Nutrition Program, The Pennsylvania State University, University Park, PA 16802

Associations Between Physical Activity and Coronary Heart Disease

Since the late 1960s, the incidence of coronary heart disease
(CHD) has decreased in the United States (1). The Surgeon General
has attributed this decline to major changes in lifestyle made by
Americans (2). Specifically, fewer people smoke, more people
monitor their blood pressure and daily stress, many have adopted
leaner diets that are lower in cholesterol and saturated fat, and
more Americans are participating in daily exercise. According to
the results of a Gallup Poll, twice as many Americans reported
exercising daily in 1977 as in 1960 (3). Currently, it is
estimated that 27-30 million Americans jog a minimum of 1-3 miles
weekly, and approximately one-half of American adults report
participating in some form of exercise daily.

The association between occupational and leisure time
physical activity and the incidence of CHD has been recognized
since the early 1950s. The incidence of fatal ischemic heart
disease (IHD) was two times greater in the professional and
business classes than in unskilled workers in Great Britian (4).
Bus drivers (who have a low level of occupational physical
activity) had a higher incidence of mortality from IHD than
conductors (who had a higher level of occupational physical
activity) (5). Ten years later it was reported that postal clerks
had higher death rates from IHD than mail carriers (6,7). Other
studies published throughout the 1960s, however, failed to show a
relationship between occupational physical activity and IHD (8-10).

Studies published during the 1950s and 1960s that examined
the relationship between occupational physical activity and CHD
were generally not designed to assess leisure time physical
activity. The failure to account for activity during leisure time
probably explains the disparate findings of these epidemiological
studies. However, in three recent studies, where occupational and
leisure time physical activity were both assessed, exercise was
associated with a lower incidence of CHD (11-13).

In the Framingham study, a prospective investigation was done
examining the relationship between level of physical activity and
mortality due to cardiovascular disease (CVD) and IHD.

0097–6156/86/0294–0059$06.25/0

Approximately 2,000 men and 2,000 women completed a questionnaire designed to assess their level of physical activity. They were studied for fourteen years and were observed for the manifestations of CVD. Death due to CVD, IHD, and all other causes decreased in men as their physical activity increased. After age and associated cardiovascular risk factors were taken into account, however, the relationship of physical activity to overall mortality persisted but was diminished. Kannel and Sorlie (11) reported a similar relationship between physical activity and mortality due to CVD and IHD in men when other risk factors were considered. In women, however, while there was a statistically significant relationship between physical activity and mortality due to CVD, this association disappeared when an adjustment was made for age and other risk factors. The authors concluded that exercise is indeed a protective factor against death from coronary disease, but its impact is not as strong as other risk factors.

Cross-Sectional and Longitudinal Studies on Healthy Subjects, Persons with Hyperlipidemia and Survivors of a Myocardial Infarct

Recognition of a beneficial effect of exercise on the incidence of CHD has led to numerous cross-sectional and longitudinal studies designed to examine the influence of physical activity on major coronary risk factors, with particular emphasis on plasma lipids and lipoproteins. A number of comprehensive reviews have summarized these studies (14-18). In general, in cross-sectional studies, high density lipoprotein (HDL) cholesterol is elevated (14) and total plasma and very low density lipoprotein (VLDL) triglycerides are lower in endurance trained subjects than in sedentary control subjects (14). In a study of 23 top-level male athletes, Lehtonen and Viikari (19) found a statistically significant relationship between the number of kilometers that the athletes ran or skied weekly and their plasma HDL cholesterol concentration (P<0.05; r=0.554). Low density lipoprotein (LDL) cholesterol is frequently lower, and plasma total cholesterol is inconsistently lower in trained subjects (19).

Despite the relatively large number of cross-sectional studies that have been reported, few have utilized women as subjects. HDL cholesterol concentration is relatively high in young sedentary women, and only vigorous rather than moderate exercise will lead to a further elevation (Table I) (20). In middle-aged women, an exercise program of moderate intensity has been associated with an elevated HDL cholesterol (21). In middle-aged men, exercise of moderate intensity is associated with greater changes in HDL cholesterol than a similar exercise program in age-matched women (21,22). Reasons for the difference in response between males and females are unidentified and deserve further investigation. Moreover, experiments designed to understand why young and middle-aged women respond differently to an exercise program of moderate intensity are needed.

From 1955 through 1981, 66 longitudinal studies were published, and from 1982 to the present, the literature in this area is voluminous (for a comprehensive review see reference 17).

Interestingly, a wide variety of experimental designs has been
employed, varying subjects (age and gender), initial and final
levels of physical fitness, and training programs
(intensity, time per session, number of weekly sessions, and
length of the program).

Tran and co-workers (17) integrated and analyzed data
collected between 1955 and 1983 and quantitatively defined the
relationships between exercise, and lipids and lipoproteins. The
data base used for their study represented 2,925 subjects (2,086
experimental subjects and 839 controls) from 66 studies. They
found that total plasma and LDL cholesterol, total triglycerides,
and the ratio of total cholesterol/HDL cholesterol were
significantly decreased, and HDL cholesterol was insignificantly
increased by exercise (Table II). They also found strong
correlations between initial total cholesterol, total
triglycerides, HDL cholesterol, and the total cholesterol/HDL
cholesterol ratio, and their respective changes as a result of
exercise. Higher initial levels of total cholesterol,
triglycerides, and total cholesterol/HDL cholesterol were
associated with the greatest decreases with exercise. Lower
initial levels of HDL cholesterol resulted in higher levels
following the exercise program. Thus, those with more 'fit'
plasma lipid profiles responded less to an exercise program than
those with 'sedentary' lipid profiles.

Longitudinal studies with young women have demonstrated that
an exercise program of moderate intensity has no effect on plasma
lipids (23,24). In one study (25), a ten-week bicycle ergometer
exercise program at 70% maximum heart rate for 30 minutes three
times weekly did not lead to changes in HDL cholesterol and
triglycerides in young (19-29 years) women. In middle-aged (35-55
years) women, however, an eight week exercise program of moderate
intensity favorably altered plasma lipids and lipoproteins; plasma
cholesterol decreased and HDL cholesterol increased (26).

Thus, while an exercise program of moderate intensity does
not significantly affect plasma lipids in young women, it appears
to favorably affect blood lipids in middle-aged women. In
physically fit and very active women (ages 23-37 years), additional
exercise (increasing the miles run weekly from 13.5 to 44.9) still
affects blood lipids (HDL cholesterol increases) (27). Further
investigations are needed to define the intensity of the exercise
program that changes the plasma lipid profile of women of varying
ages.

Exercise has been shown to reduce (28), and in some studies
normalize (29,30) plasma triglyceride concentrations in persons
with hypertriglyceridemia. In persons with hypercholesterolemia,
plasma triglycerides and HDL cholesterol correlated with physical
activity; the most physically active men had the lowest plasma
triglyceride and highest HDL cholesterol concentrations (31).
Survivors of a myocardial infarct also have favorable changes in
their blood lipid profile in response to exercise of moderate
intensity (32-36).

It will be important to determine whether the positive effects
of exercise slow the progression or perhaps lead to a reversal of
existing atherosclerosis.

Table I. Exercise Intensity and HDL Cholesterol in Females[a]

Sport	Age	Exercise Intensity	HDL-cholesterol
	years		mg/dl
Swimming[b]	19-22	sedentary	67.2 ± 14.0^d
		moderate	70.0 ± 10.9^d
		high	82.0 ± 14.6^e
Long Distance Running/Jogging[c]	24-58	sedentary	62.0 ± 13.4^d
		moderate	70.0 ± 21.8^e
		high	78.0 ± 16.6^f

[a] $\overline{X} \pm SD$
[d,e,f] Means in the same column within a group (sport) not sharing a common superscript are significantly different ($P<0.05$).
[b] Smith et al. (20)
[c] Moore et al. (21)

Table II. Overall Changes in Plasma Lipids and Lipoproteins Following an Exercise Program

Total Cholesterol	*< 10 mg/dl	$P < 0.01$
Total Triglycerides	< 15.8 mg/dl	$P < 0.01$
HDL Cholesterol	> 1.2 mg/dl	NS[a]
LDL Cholesterol	< 5.1 mg/dl	$P < 0.05$
Total Cholesterol HDL Cholesterol	< 0.48	$P < 0.01$

NOTE: There were no changes in the controls.

Reproduced with permission from Ref. 17. Copyright 1983 American College of Sports Medicine.

NS = Not significant
*< decreased
 > increased

Factors Affecting Plasma Lipids and Lipoproteins with Exercise

Numerous factors affect plasma lipids and lipoproteins, and some investigators have attempted to control for these variables in designing studies to assess the effect of exercise on plasma lipids.   Tran et al. (17) identified six variables that affected the results of longitudinal studies designed to assess the relationship between exercise and plasma lipids.   These variables were age, sex, intensity of the exercise program, VO_2 max achieved, body weight and changes in body weight, and changes in percent body fat (Table III).   There is evidence that failure to control for these variables may be responsible for the inconsistent findings of studies designed to examine the relationship between exercise and lipoproteins (37).

Williams et al. (37) found that the decrease in body weight due to exercise was associated with an increase in plasma HDL cholesterol concentration in middle-aged men.   They suggested that processes associated with weight change may produce many, but not all, of the changes in HDL cholesterol that had been previously associated with exercise.

In a cross-sectional study involving marathon runners, Willett et al. (38) used multiple regression to determine the effects that age, weight, height, average number of miles run per week and best marathon time had on the relationship between alcohol consumption and HDL cholesterol.   Alcohol consumption was associated with an increase in HDL cholesterol beyond the increase related to physical activity.

A number of dietary factors have been shown to influence HDL cholesterol concentrations (39-42), and some investigators have attempted to control for diet in their analysis of exercise and plasma lipid relationships (22,43).   Hartung et al. (22) found no major dietary differences between distance runners and a sedentary control group and concluded that differences in HDL cholesterol concentrations between groups were likely due to exercise.   Blair and colleagues (43) reported a higher intake of total fat, carbohydrates, and kilocalories in distance runners than in the sedentary control group, but the percent distribution of macronutrients was similar between groups.   The authors also concluded that differences in HDL cholesterol concentrations between groups were unlikely due to dietary differences.   In a cross-sectional study involving distance runners and a sedentary control group, Thompson et al. (44) reported that runners consumed significantly more kilocalories and carbohydrates than sedentary controls and concluded that differences in the lipoprotein profile of athletes may be related, in part, to diet; however, this study did not include a statistical analysis of the effect of diet on exercise and plasma lipid relationships.

In a study involving young male and female college students, in which diet and body weight remained constant during a six-week exercise conditioning program, there was no change in HDL cholesterol (45).   Lipson et al. (45) suggested that exercise-induced changes in HDL cholesterol concentration found in other studies may be mediated, in part, by uncontrolled variables such as changes in diet, body weight, and life-style.

Table III.   Impact of Factors Affecting Plasma Lipids and
            Lipoproteins with Exercise

Plasma Lipid/ Lipoprotein	Factor	Change in Lipid/Lipoprotein
Total Cholesterol HDL Cholesterol Total Triglycerides	Age	Larger decreases in older subjects
HDL Cholesterol LDL Cholesterol	Age and sex	Larger changes in older males
All Lipids and Lipoproteins	Intensity	More beneficial changes at an exercise program of lower intensity (must be at least 60% of maximum heart rate) of longer duration
Total Cholesterol	VO_2 Max	Larger decreases with larger increases in VO_2 max
HDL Cholesterol	VO_2	Larger increases with larger increases in VO_2 max
Total Triglycerides Total Cholesterol LDL Cholesterol	Body weight	Those with higher initial body weights and the greatest decrease in body weight had the greatest decreases
Total Cholesterol HDL Cholesterol LDL Cholesterol	%Body fat	Greater decreases with greater decreases in % body fat
HDL Cholesterol	% Body fat	Greater increases with greater decreases in % body fat

Reproduced with permission from Ref. 17.   Copyright 1983 American
College of Sports Medicine.

In a well-controlled study designed to assess the influence of the type and amount of dietary lipid on plasma lipid concentrations in endurance athletes, Lukaski et al. (46) reported that the plasma response to dietary lipid was not attenuated in men who were physically very active. In contrast, Quig and associates (47) reported that plasma total cholesterol concentration was lower in subjects who exercised and who ate a diet containing 0.4 or 1.4 gm of cholesterol daily. Thus, the influence of diet on the relationship between exercise and plasma lipids remains equivocal.

Subjects' gender also affects results of studies designed to examine exercise and plasma lipid relationships. Tran and associates (17) reported a significant relationship between initial and final plasma total cholesterol and triglycerides in males but not in females, and a significant relationship between initial and final HDL cholesterol and the ratio of total cholesterol/HDL cholesterol in both males and females. Accordingly, exercise had relatively less significance in influencing the ratio of HDL cholesterol/total cholesterol in females than males (48); for females a number of other factors were relatively more significant.

Gender-related differences in exercise-induced changes in plasma lipids may be related to a number of factors (25,48), one of which appears to be sex hormone concentrations (49). Following a ten-week bicycle exercise training study, testosterone, total testosterone (including dihydrotestosterone), and estrone were significantly and positively correlated with HDL cholesterol in 12 men (18-32 years) (49). In addition, the change in both total testosterone and testosterone was also positively correlated with the change in HDL cholesterol with exercise (49). Testosterone concentration fell while estrogen concentration rose with exercise (49). Others have shown that exogenous estrogen increases HDL cholesterol in women, (50) and Frey and co-workers (49) suggested that the exercise-induced changes in testosterone and estrogen may mediate changes in plasma lipids and lipoproteins with exercise.

Differences in the activity of lipoprotein lipase (LPL) between men and women may explain, in part, the different plasma lipid response to exercise (48). The activity of adipose tissue LPL is higher in women than in men, and higher in sedentary women than in male long distance runners (51). Since the intra-vascular production of HDL is augmented by the catabolism of triglyceride rich lipoproteins by LPL (52), this hypothesis deserves further attention.

Mechanisms of Exercise-Induced Changes in Plasma Lipids: Lipoprotein Lipase, Hepatic Triglyceride Lipase and Lecithin Cholesterol Acyl Transferase

There has been considerable interest in elucidating the mechanisms by which exercise leads to reciprocal changes in plasma HDL cholesterol and triglycerides. To date, most studies have been designed to identify changes that occur with exercise--changes in the activities of enzymes such as LPL, hepatic triglyceride lipase (HL), and lecithin cholesterol acyl transferase (LCAT). In addition, investigators have studied the effects of exercise on triglyceride production and hepatic lipoprotein production in the rat.

LPL is located on the endothelial surface of capillaries in muscle and adipose tissue (53). This enzyme degrades triglyceride-rich lipoproteins to free fatty acids and 2-monoglyceride (53). Following isomerization to 1-monoglyceride and lipolysis to free fatty acids and glyceride, the free fatty acids are then taken up by skeletal muscle and adipose tissue and oxidized for energy or used for triglyceride deposition. During prolonged exercise, free fatty acids are a major fuel source for muscle (54).

Hepatic lipase (HL), which is present on the endothelial cells of liver sinusoids (55), preferentially hydrolyzes phosphatidylcholine in HDL_2, and the product is removed with esterified and unesterified cholesterol by the liver (56). Although the precise function of HL is unknown, it has been implicated recently in the metabolism/catabolism of HDL_2 by the liver with the subsequent generation of a more dense HDL subfraction, HDL_3 (57).

LCAT promotes the transfer of fatty acids from the 2-position of lecithin to unesterified cholesterol in nascent HDL (58,59). Hence, discoidal nascent HDL are converted to mature spherical particles via the enzymatic action of LCAT. In addition, LCAT affects the net movement of cholesterol from peripheral tissues to the liver and/or to other lipoproteins for catabolism (60,61) and facilitates the removal of cholesterol from the plasma (62).

In a comprehensive investigation designed to study the relationship between the activity of LPL and HDL, Nikkila and associates (51) reported that male champion-class long-distance runners had elevated skeletal muscle and adipose tissue LPL activities versus sedentary subjects. Only skeletal muscle LPL activity was elevated in female runners. Whole body LPL activity was estimated to be 2.3 and 1.5 times higher in male and female runners, respectively, and all athletes had higher HDL cholesterol concentrations than the sedentary control groups; however, plasma and lipoprotein cholesterol and triglycerides were not different. Adipose tissue LPL activity was positively correlated (r=0.94) with HDL cholesterol when the values for all groups (males, females, athletes, sedentary controls), including an additional group of male sprinters, were used in the analysis.

The activity of LPL in adipose tissue of 20 middle-aged males (31-49 years) was 56% higher following their participation in a fifteen-week exercise program that consisted of at least three 30-60 minute exercise bouts per week (63). The experimental subjects also had a 7% increase in HDL cholesterol, an insignificant decrease in total plasma cholesterol, a significant decrease in LDL cholesterol, and a 33% elevation in postheparin plasma LPL activity (which includes both LPL and HL). Although plasma triglycerides did not decrease with exercise, there was a strong negative association between HDL cholesterol and plasma triglyceride concentration before and after the exercise program.

In response to exercise there are significant increases in postheparin and adipose tissue LPL activity concomitant with changes in plasma lipids. These synchronous changes in LPL activity and plasma lipids and lipoproteins are suggestive of a possible relationship between both.

Components of triglyceride--rich lipoproteins undergoing lipolysis appear to be incorporated into discordal nascent HDL particles by a number of different mechanisms (52). The subsequent metabolism of these particles via the interaction of LCAT with free cholesterol derived from cell membranes or other lipoproteins leads to the formation of mature HDL particles (Figure 1). With an increase in the activity of LPL with exercise, it is hypothesized that the catabolism of triglyceride-rich lipoproteins is enhanced, leading to an increased formation of HDL (Figure 1). Associated with this increase in triglyceride hydrolysis is a concommitant decrease in plasma triglyceride. Thus, the effect of exercise on LPL provides a mechanism which results in an increase in HDL and conversely a decrease in plasma triglycerides. This proposed mechanism is yet highly speculative but worthy of further attention.

Plasma HDL_2 cholesterol was positively correlated with physical fitness and inversely correlated with HL activity in young men (64), and HL activity was lower in 20 middle-aged men who completed an exercise program of moderate intensity for fifteen weeks (65). In addition, postheparin plasma HL activity was significantly and negatively correlated with HDL cholesterol before and after the exercise program ($r=-0.50$) (86). These findings have been confirmed by other studies (66,67).

The hypothesized mechanism by which a decrease in HL activity leads to an increase in HDL cholesterol, or the HDL_2 subfraction, is illustrated in figure 2. As HL activity decreases, less HDL_2 is metabolized/catabolized by the liver, leading to an increase in the concentration of this particle in the plasma. This mechanism is as yet speculative.

Exercise leads to an increase in the activity of LCAT (68). At the end of a fifteen-week aerobic exercise program, 19 male participants had a 14% increase in physical performance capacity and a twofold increase in LCAT activity (68). LCAT activity was elevated after seven weeks of exercise, and it continued to increase significantly throughout the remainder of the exercise program. At present, however, the magnitude of the effect of exercise on LCAT activity is not clear.

A proposed mechanism by which an exercise-induced increase in LCAT leads to an increase in HDL cholesterol is illustrated in figure 3. An increase in both Apo AI and LCAT activity in response to exercise could lead to increased esterification of cholesterol in HDL and thereby allows for an increase in the transport of free cholesterol from tissues and other lipoproteins to nascent HDL, and enhanced formation of HDL_2. While still speculative, this proposed mechanism deserves attention.

At present, the mechanism (5) of the exercise-induced changes in plasma lipids and lipoproteins is/are undefined. While significant attention in this section has been directed toward understanding the roles of various enzymes in lipoprotein production, catabolism and metabolism with exercise, no definite information is available to support the hypotheses raised. An alternative, yet highly viable possibility includes simply the availability of substrate which may well exist in considerable excess or substrate activity of relevant lipoprotein particles

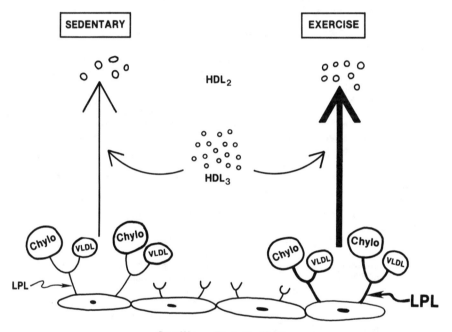

Figure 1. Proposed yet speculative mechanism by which
high-density lipoprotein (HDL) increases in response to
exercise via increased lipoprotein lipase (LPL) activity.
During lipolysis, components of Tg-rich lipoproteins are
transferred to and incorporated into HDL_3 leading to the
formation of HDL_2. Very low density lipoprotein (VLDL),
chylomicron (chylo).

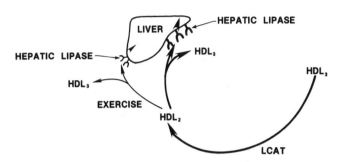

Figure 2. Proposed yet speculative mechanism by which high-density lipoprotein (HDL) increases in response to exercise via decreased hepatic lipase activity. Lecithin cholesterol acyl transferase (LCAT).

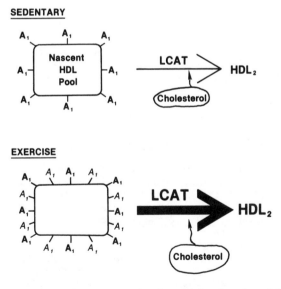

Figure 3. Proposed yet speculative mechanism by which high-density lipoprotein (HDL) increases in response to exercise via increased lecithin cholesterol acyl transferase (LCAT) activity and/or increased apolipoprotein A_1 concentration.

which in turn may profoundly regulate the enzymatic reactions discussed. Clearly, a great deal of work is needed in this area to clarify the role(s) of LPL, HL and LCAT in changing plasma lipids and lipoproteins in response to exercise.

Hepatic Triglyceride Production and Extrahepatic Triglyceride Removal

Although it is generally recognized that exercise decreases plasma triglyceride concentrations, the mechanism(s) by which this occurs are not clear. Simonelli and Eaton (69) found that a three-week program of voluntary wheel running resulted in a 51% decrease in triglyceride secretion in exercised versus sedentary rats. They also found that an exogenous lipid load was cleared more quickly by obese exercised versus obese sedentary rats.

A decreased triglyceride secretion with exercise has also been reported by Dall'Aglio and associates (70); however, the magnitude of the decrease could not be accounted for by a decrease just in hepatic production. The results of this study indicate that both extrahepatic and hepatic mechanisms are involved in the exercise-induced reduction of plasma triglycerides.

We have found that exercised obese Zucker, lean Zucker, and Fischer 344 rats had lower plasma triglycerides than sedentary rats (71,72) (Tables IV and V). In Zucker rats this was due to a lower chylomicron triglyceride concentration. Hepatic VLDL triglyceride production, measured via a recycled in situ liver perfusion technique, did not differ between exercised and sedentary rats of each phenotype (data not shown). This suggests extrahepatic mechanisms are predominant in the hypotriglyceridemic action of exercise.

In summary, evidence indicates that both hepatic and extrahepatic mechanisms are involved in the exercise-induced decrease of plasma triglycerides. Differences in the methods used to assess triglyceride production rates may explain, in part, disparate findings. Further investigations are needed to define the role of the liver and extrahepatic sites in the production and catabolism of triglycerides with exercise.

Hepatic Lipid and Lipoprotein Production

Few investigators have examined hepatic lipid and lipoprotein production in response to exercise. Because nascent HDL are synthesized in the liver, intestine, and the plasma via the catabolism of triglyceride rich lipoproteins (52), exercise-induced modifications in any or all of these systems could lead to changes in the plasma lipoprotein profile.

Seelbach and Kris-Etherton (72) recently examined the effect of a vigorous ten-week exercise program on hepatic lipoprotein cholesterol and triglyceride production in obese and lean Zucker rats. (The obese Zucker rat has a marked hyperlipidemia with elevations of all plasma lipoprotein fractions, and the lean Zucker rat has a plasma lipoprotein profile similar to that of other lean rats. The use of both lean and obese strains provides information on the effect of exercise on hepatic lipoprotein production and

Table IV. Plasma and Lipoprotein Triglyceride Concentrations in Zucker Rats[a]

	Obese		Lean	
	Sedentary	Runners	Sedentary	Runners
		mg/dl		
Plasma Triglycerides	335 ± 36^b	177 ± 32^c	116 ± 10^d	71 ± 10^e
Chylomicron	216 ± 46^b	73 ± 8^c	54 ± 13^c	15 ± 6^d
VLDL	$46 \pm 10^{b,c}$	51 ± 19^b	$32 \pm 6^{b,c}$	19 ± 3^c

[a]Values represent $\bar{x} \pm$ SEM.
[b,c,d,e]Means in the same row not sharing a common superscript are significantly different (P<0.05).
Data from Ref. 72.

Table V. Plasma Triglyceride Concentration in Fisher 344 Rats[a]

Treatment	Plasma Triglyceride (mg/dl)
Normocholesterolemic Diet + Sedentary	380 ± 165^b
Hypercholesterolemic Diet + Exercise	156 ± 103^c
Hypercholesterolemic Diet + Sedentary	365 ± 155^b

[a]Values represent mean ±S.D.
[b,c]Means with different superscripts are different (P<0.05).
Data from Ref. 71.

plasma lipoproteins in both a normal and a hyperlipidemic state.)
Weanling rats, twenty-eight days old, were exercised on a
motor-driven treadmill at a speed of 0.8 mph at an 8% grade for 90
minutes per day, six days a week for ten weeks. Hepatic HDL
cholesterol production was significantly higher in lean Zucker
runners compared with all other groups (Table VI). Hepatic HDL
cholesterol production tended to be lower in obese runners, but
there was considerable individual variation among animals, and
differences between obese sedentary and exercised rats failed to
reach statistical significance (Table VI). Exercise had no effect
on hepatic VLDL and LDL cholesterol production secretion in either
obese or lean rats. These results are the first to demonstrate an
effect of vigorous exercise on hepatic HDL cholesterol production.
It is interesting to note that exercise affected hepatic HDL
cholesterol production differently in obese and lean Zucker rats.

In this study, both groups of exercised animals had lower
plasma total cholesterol and chylomicron cholesterol than
appropriate sedentary control animals (Table VI). Unexpectedly,
plasma HDL cholesterol was also lower in both groups of exercised
animals (Table VI). Together with the results obtained on hepatic
HDL cholesterol production, these data demonstrate that plasma HDL
cholesterol concentration reflects hepatic HDL cholesterol
production in obese, but not in lean rats.

Mela and Kris-Etherton (71) recently characterized the plasma
lipoprotein profile and assessed hepatic lipoprotein cholesterol
production in exercised Fischer 344 rats fed either a
hypercholesterolemic or normocholesterolemic diet. Weanling rats
were assigned to one of three experimental treatments: 1) rats
were fed a semisynthetic hypercholesterolemic diet containing 10%
lard and 0.4% cholesterol and exercised for ten weeks, six days per
week, for one hour daily at 1.2-1.4 km/hr at a 9% grade; 2) rats
were fed the same diet and remained sedentary; 3) rats were fed a
normocholesterolemic diet (no lard or cholesterol added) and
remained sedentary. The three groups are referred to as HE
(hyperlipemic diet + exercise), HS (hyperlipemic diet + sedentary),
and NS (normolipemic diet + sedentary). Hepatic HDL cholesterol
production was higher in NS than HS rats with values for HE rats in
between and not significantly different from the other two groups
(Table VII). In these experiments there was a trend for hepatic
HDL cholesterol production to increase in response to exercise. In
addition, exercise had an ameliorative effect on diet-induced
changes in hepatic HDL cholesterol production.

Total plasma cholesterol was higher in both HE and HS rats
than in NS rats. However, HE rats had a lower plasma total
cholesterol concentration than HS rats (Table VII). Plasma HDL
cholesterol was higher in NS than in HS rats with values for HE
rats in between and not significantly different from the other two
groups. Thus, in contrast to results reported for lean Zucker
rats, the plasma HDL cholesterol concentration reflected hepatic
HDL cholesterol production in Fischer 344 rats fed a
hypercholesterolemic diet. Plasma VLDL cholesterol was higher in
rats fed the hypercholesterolemic diet but was unaffected by
exercise (Table VII), and LDL cholesterol was similar among groups
(data not shown). In this experiment, exercise ameliorated some of
the diet-induced changes in plasma lipids.

Table VI. Plasma Total, Chylomicron, and HDL Cholesterol and Hepatic HDL Cholesterol Production in Lean and Obese Zucker Rats in Response to Exercise[a]

	Obese		Lean	
	Sedentary	Runners	Sedentary	Runners
	mg/dl			
Plasma Total Cholesterol	80.4±3.1[b]	66.1±4.0[c]	57.0±1.0[d]	49.3±1.2[e]
Chylomicron	9.9±0.8[b]	3.5±0.5[c]	4.6±0.4[c]	1.9±0.3[d]
HDL	54.9±2.4[b]	40.2±2.1[c]	37.3±0.6[c]	32.6±0.8[d]
	ug/gm liver/hr			
Hepatic HDL Cholesterol Production	9.5±1.0[b]	8.3±1.0[b]	11.2±1.1[b]	17.0±1.1[c]

[a] Values are $\bar{x}$ ± SEM
[b,c,d,e] Means in the same row not sharing a common superscript are significantly different ($P<0.05$).
Data from ref. 72.

Table VII. Plasma Total, VLDL, and HDL Cholesterol and Hepatic HDL Cholesterol Production in Fischer 344 Rats in Response to Exercise[a]

	Hypercholes- terolemic Diet + Sedentary	Hypercholes- terolemic Diet + Exercise	Normocholes- terolemic Diet + Sedentary
	mg/dl		
Plasma Total Cholesterol	98.8 ± 16.8[b]	71.4 ± 13.8[c]	58.8 ± 5.4[d]
VLDL Cholesterol	8.3 ± 3.9[b]	9.0 ± 2.8[b]	< 1[b,c]
HDL Cholesterol	23.1 ± 3.0[b]	24.4 ± 3.3[b,c]	25.6 ± 2.8[c]
	ug/gm liver/hr		
Hepatic HDL Cholesterol Production	4.76 ± 2.42[a]	6.14 ± 1.95[a,b]	9.44 ± 4.12[b]

[a] Values are $\bar{x}$ ± SD.
[b,c,d] Means in the same row not sharing a common superscript are significantly different ($P<0.05$).
Data from Ref. 71.

In summary, it appears that hepatic HDL cholesterol production
is altered with exercise. Factors such as adiposity and diet, and
others that are as yet unidentified, may mask the detection of
changes in HDL cholesterol production with exercise.

The Effect of Exercise on Cholesterol Metabolism

A number of investigators have demonstrated a marked reduction in
hepatic cholesterol concentration in exercised rats (73-75). In
Fischer 344 rats, liver cholesterol was 30% lower in exercised rats
than in sedentary rats when both were fed a mildly
hypercholesterolemic diet (71). However, exercised rats still had
an elevated liver cholesterol concentration compared to sedentary
rats fed a normocholesterolemic diet suggesting that exercise does
not normalize diet induced elevations in hepatic cholesterol
concentration (71).

An increased cholesterol excretion, degradation, and decreased
synthesis may explain the lower hepatic cholesterol concentration
reported in exercised versus sedentary rats. In support of the
former, Gollnick and Simmons (73) reported that exercised rats
excreted significantly more fecal sterol than sedentary rats.
Others have reported similar findings (76-78) as well as an
increased degradation of cholesterol in exercised mice and an
increased duodenal bile flow and biliary cholesterol excretion in
subjects following only 30 minutes of cycling.

Diet or exercise had no effect on carcass cholesterol
concentration in Fischer 344 rats fed a hypercholesterolemic diet
(71). However, total carcass cholesterol tended to be lower in
exercised rats than in sedentary rats. Carcass cholesterol
concentration was similar between exercised and sedentary rats, but
the body weights of sedentary rats were higher. Both sedentary and
exercised rats fed the hypercholesterolemic diet had equivalent
food, and hence cholesterol intakes. These data suggest that
exercise increases cholesterol excretion and/or degradation, or
decreases cholesterol synthesis in the rat.

Effect of Exercise on the Development and Progression of Atherosclerosis

Direct proof of a protective effect of exercise on the development
of atherosclerosis in humans is lacking. To date, only a few
animal studies have provided strong evidence in favor of a
beneficial effect of exercise on diet-induced atherogenesis
(79,80).

Kramsch and co-workers (79) examined the effect of exercise on
plasma lipids and lipoproteins and the development of
atherosclerosis in nonhuman primates. Nine Macaca fascicularis
monkeys remained sedentary and were fed a control diet. A second
group remained sedentary and was fed a control diet for twelve
months followed by the control diet plus 0.1% cholesterol and 10%
butter (atherogenic diet) for twenty-four months. A third group
was fed the control diet for eighteen months followed by the
atherogenic diet for twenty-four months. When animals in the third
group were approximately 1 year of age, they were gradually

conditioned to treadmill exercise over a twelve month period and
then kept physically active for an additional six months.
Thereafter, the exercise program was maintained and the monkeys
were fed the atherogenic diet for twenty-four months. At the end
of the study, both sedentary and exercised monkeys fed the
atherogenic diet had elevations in VLDL and LDL cholesterol, and
plasma cholesterol concentrations were significantly higher than
those of sedentary animals fed the control diet (620 vs 100 mg/dl).
Plasma HDL cholesterol concentration, however, was higher in
exercised than sedentary monkeys. Of major significance was the
finding that exercised monkeys had significantly less
atherosclerotic disease than sedentary monkeys.

Hasler et al. (80) have recently shown that a vigorous
exercise markedly retards the development of atherosclerosis in
Fischer 344 rats fed an atherogenic diet. While there were no
grossly visible atherosclerotic plaques present in exercised or
sedentary rats, microscopic sections of the abdominal aorta were
markedly different between exercised and sedentary animals. Aortas
of sedentary rats fed a diet with 10% lard, 0.4% cholesterol had a
high degree of plaque development, fat accumulation,
mineralization, erosion, and necrosis. Exercised rats fed the same
diet had less atherosclerotic involvement. Specifically, there was
only moderate rather than severe intimal proliferation, subintimal
plaque formation, and fiber degeneration in exercised versus
sedentary rats. Eighty percent of the exercised animals had a
mildly irregular aortic intimal surface, and none had marked
erosion, whereas 80% of the sedentary animals had a moderate to
marked aortic intimal surface erosion. Link et al. (81) also found
significant differences in the extent of atherosclerosis between
exercised and sedentary swine fed an atherogenic diet. Exercise
has also been shown to decrease the severity of experimentally
induced atherosclerosis in ducks (82), geese (82,83), and rabbits
(84-87).

The studies that have shown a beneficial effect of exercise in
retarding the development of atherosclerosis in swine and nonhuman
primates suggest a beneficial effect in humans. This, of course,
awaits confirmation. Of equal importance, as well, is the need for
well-controlled investigations to assess the effect of exercise on
the reversal of existing atherosclerosis.

Summary

Although coronary heart disease (CHD) is still the leading cause of
death in the United States, there has been a considerable decrease
since the late 1960s. The Surgeon General has attributed this
decline to lifestyle changes that Americans have made.
Specifically, fewer people smoke, more people monitor their blood
pressure and daily stress, many have adopted leaner diets that are
lower in cholesterol, and more Americans are exercising. In fact,
in 1977, one-half of all American adults reported participating in
daily physical activity.

The association between the lack of physical activity and the
incidence of CHD has been recognized since the 1950s. Studies have
shown that persons who participate in some form of physical

activity have less coronary disease and fewer fatal heart attacks
than sedentary persons.

Exercise may exert a beneficial effect on one's risk of CHD by
altering blood lipids. High density lipoprotein cholesterol, both
a vehicle for cholesterol transport in the blood and a particle
that confers protection against CHD, is increased with exercise.
An exercise program of moderate intensity (jogging for 20 minutes,
3 times a week) leads to beneficial changes in blood lipids in
middle-aged women (but not in young women) and in men and survivors
of a heart attack. Vigorous exercise is necessary to beneficially
affect blood lipids in young women.

Exercise is effective in ameliorating the development of
atherosclerosis in exercised animals fed a high fat, high
cholesterol diet. While it has not been unequivocally demonstrated
that exercise retards the development of atherosclerosis in humans,
participation in a program of regular exercise may decrease one's
risk of developing CHD.

Acknowledgments

I wish to thank Dr. Terry Etherton, Lee Alekel, Richard Cohen,
Clare Hasler, Debra Krummel, D.J. Mela, and Shiromi Padmanathan for
helpful suggestions in the preparation of this review. In
addition, the assistance of Tamara Snyder, Lisa Bates, Mary Alice
Gettings, Fred VandenHeede, and Nancy Hopkins is appreciated.

Literature Cited

1.   Levy, R.I. Arteriosclerosis 1981, 1, 312-25.
2.   Richmond, J.B., Surgeon General. Dallas Times Herald
     interview, May 26, 1980. pg. column.
3.   The Gallup Poll: Public Opinion 1972-1977; Vol. 2:
     1200-1202, Scholarly Resources, Inc., Wilmington, Delaware,
     1978.
4.   Logan, W.P.D. Lancet 1952, 1, 758.
5.   Morris, J.N., Heady, J.A., Raffle, P.A.B., Roberts, L.G., and
     Parks, J.W. Lancet, 1953 265:1053-1057, 1111-1120.
6.   Morris, J.N. Cardiol. Prat. 1962, 13, 85-95.
7.   Kahn, H.A. Am. J. Public Health 1963, 53, 1058-67.
8.   Paul, O., Lepper, M.H., Phelan, W.H., Dupertuis, G.W.,
     MacMillan, A., McKean, H., and Park, H. Circulation 1963, 28,
     20-31.
9.   Chapman, J.M. and Massey, F.J., Jr. J. Chronic Dis. 1964, 17,
     933-49.
10. Taylor, H.L. Can. Med. Assoc. J. 1967, 96, 825-31.
11. Kannel, W.B. and Sorlie, P. Arch. Internal Med. 1979, 139,
     857-861.
12. Morris, J.N., Pollard, R., Everitt, M.G., Chave, S.P.W.
     Lancet 1980, 2, 1207-10.
13. Paffenbarger, R.S., Wing, A.L., and Hyde, R.T. Am. J. Epidem.
     1978, 108, 161-75.
14. Dufaux, B., Assman, G., and Hollman, W. Int. J. Sports Med.
     1982, 3, 123-36.

15. Huttunen, J.K. Ann. Clin. Res. 1982, 14, Suppl. 34, 124-9.
16. Moffat, R.J. and Gilliam, T.B. Artery 1979, 6, 1-19.
17. Tran, Z.V., Weltman, A., Glass, G.V., and Mood, D.P. Med. Sci. Sports Exer. 1983, 15, 393-402.
18. Wood, P.D. and Haskell, W.L. Lipids 1979, 14, 417-27.
19. Lehtonen, A. and Viikari, J. Acta Med. Scand. 1978, 204, 111-4.
20. Smith, M.P., Mendez, J., Druckenmiller, M., and Kris-Etherton, P.M. Am. J. Clin. Nutr. 1982, 36, 251-5.
21. Moore, C.E., Hartung, G.H., Mitchell, R.E., Kappus, C.M., and Hinderlitter, J. Metabolism 1983, 32, 189-96.
22. Hartung, G.H., Foreyt, J.P., Mitchell, R.E., et al. N. Eng. J. Med. 1980, 302, 357-61.
23. Wynne, T.F., Frey, M.A.B., Laubach, L.L., and Glueck, C.J. Metabolism 1980, 29, 1267-71.
24. Moll, M.E., Williams, R.S., Lester, R.M., Quadfordt, S.H., and Wallace, A.G. Atherosclerosis 1979, 34, 159-66.
25. Frey, M.A.B., Doerr, B.M., Laubach, L.L., Mann, B.L., and Glueck, J. Metabolism 1982, 31, 1142-6.
26. Reid, E., Talano, C.M., Buskirk, E., Green, M., and Kris-Etherton, P.M. Submitted for publication.
27. Rotkis, T., Boyden, T.W., Pamenter, R.W., Stanforth, P., and Wilmore, J. Metabolism 1981, 30, 994-5.
28. Gyntelberg, F., Brennan, R., Holloszy, J.O., Schonfeld, G., Rennie, M.J., and Weidman, S.W. Am. J. Clin. Nutr. 1977, 30, 716-20.
29. Oscai, L.B., Patterson, J.A., Bogard, D.L., Beck, R.J., and Rothermel, B.L. Am. J. Cardiology 1972, 30, 775-80.
30. Lampman, R.M., Santinga, J.T., Hodge, M.F., Block, W.D., Flora, J.D., and Bassett, D.R. Circulation 1977, 55, 652-9.
31. Gordon, D.J., Witztum, J.L., Hunninghake, D., Gates, S., and Glueck, C.L. Circulation 1983, 67, 512-20.
32. LaRosa, J.C., Cleary, P., Muesing, R.A., Gorman, P., Hellerstein, H.K., and Naughton, J. Arch. Intern. Med. 1982, 142, 2269-74.
33. Kavanagh, T., Shephard, R.J., Lindley, L.J., and Pieper, M. Arteriosclerosis 1983, 3, 249-59.
34. Ballantyne, F.C., Clark, R.S., Simpson, H.S., and Ballantyne, D. Circulation 1982, 65, 913-8.
35. Hartung, G.H., Squires, W.G., and Gotto, A.M., Jr. Am. Heart J. 1981, 101, 181-4.
36. Streja, D. and Mymin, D. JAMA 1979, 242, 2190-2.
37. Williams, P.T., Wood, P.D., Haskell, W.L., and Vranizan, K. JAMA 1982, 247, 2674-9.
38. Willett, W., Hennekens, C.H., Siegal, A.J., Adner, M.M., and Castelli, W.P. N. Eng. J. Med. 1980, 303, 1159-61.
39. Shepard, B., Packard, C.J., Patsch, J.R., Gotto, A.M., Jr., and Taunton, O.D. J. Clin. Invest. 1978, 61, 1582-91.
40. Shonfeld, G., Weidmann, S.W., Witztum, J.L., and Bowen, R.M. Metabolism 1976, 25, 261-75.
41. Blum, C.B., Levy, R.I., Eisenberg, S., Hall, M., III, Goebel, R.H., and Berman, M. J. Clin. Invest. 1977, 60, 795-807.
42. Wilson, D.E. and Lees, R.S. J. Clin. Invest. 1972, 51, 1051-7.

43. Blair, S.N., Ellsworth, N.M., Haskell, W.L., Stern, M.P., Farquhar, J.W., and Wood, P.D. Med. Sci. Sports Exer. 1981, 13, 310-5.

44. Thompson, P.D., Lazarus, B., Cullinane, E., Henderson, L.O., Musliner, T., Eshleman, R., and Herbert, P.N. Atherosclerosis 1983, 46, 333-9.

45. Lipson, L.C., Bonow, R.O., Schaefer, E.J., Brewer, H.B., and Lindgren, F.T. Atherosclerosis 1980, 37, 529-38.

46. Lukaski, H.C., Bolonchuk, W.W., Klevay, L.M., Mahalko, J.R., Milne, D.B., and Sandstead, H.H. Am. J. Clin. Nutr. 1984, 39, 35-44.

47. Quig, D.W., Thye, F.W., Ritchey, S.J., Herbert, W.G., Clevidence, B.A., Reynolds, L.K., and Smith, M.C. Am. J. Clin. Nutr. 1983, 38, 825-34.

48. Nakamura, N., Uzawa, H., Maeda, H., and Inomoto, T. Atherosclerosis 1983, 48, 173-83.

49. Frey, M.A.B., Doerr, B.M., Srivastava, L.S., and Glueck, C.J. J. Appl. Physiol. 1983, 54, 757-62.

50. Wallace, R.B., Hoover, J., Barrett-Connor, E., Rifkind, B.M., Hunninghake, D.B., Mackenthum, G., and Heiss, G. Lancet 1979, 2, 112-5.

51. Nikkila, E.A., Taskinen, M.R., Rehumen, S., and Harkonen, M. Metabolism 1978, 27, 1661-71.

52. Tall, A. and Small, D. Adv. Lipid Res. 1980, 17, 1-51.

53. Nilsson-Ehle, P., Garfinkel, A.S., and Schotz, M.C. Ann. Rev. Biochem. 1980, 49, 667-93.

54. Havel, R.J., Naimark, A., and Borchgrevink, C.F. J. Clin. Invest. 1963, 42, 1054-63.

55. Kuusi, T., Nikkila, E.A., Virtanen, I., and Kinnunen, P.K.J. Biochem. J. 1979, 181, 245-6.

56. Groot, P.H., Jansen, H., and VanTol, A. FEBS Letters 1981, 129, 269-72.

57. Kuusi, T., Saarinen, P., and Nikkila, E.A. Atherosclerosis 1980, 36, 589-93.

58. Glomset, J.A. J. Lipid Res. 1968, 9, 155-67.

59. Glomset, J.A. Biochem. Biophys. Acta. 1962, 65, 128-35.

60. Glomset, J.A. In "The Biochem of Atherosclerosis"; Scanu, A.M., Ed.; Marcel Dekker: New York, 1979, pp. 247-73.

61. Bowden, J.A. In "High Density Lipoproteins"; Day, C.E., Ed.; Marcel Dekker: New York, 1981, pp. 149-75.

62. Glomset, J.A. In "The Biochemistry of Atherosclerosis"; Scanu, A.M., Ed.; Marcel Dekker: New York, 1979, pp. 247-73.

63. Peltonen, P., Marniemi, J., Hietanen, E., Vuori, I., and Ehnholm, C. Metabolism 1981, 30, 518-26.

64. Kuusi, T., Nikkila, E.A., Saarinen, P., Varjo, P., and Laitinen, L.A. Atherosclerosis 1982, 41, 209-19.

65. Peltonen, P., Marniemi, J., Vuori, I., and Hietanen, E. Metabolism 1981, 30, 518-26.

66. Marniemi, J., Peltonen, P., Vuori, I, and Hietanen, E. Acta. Physiol. Scand. 1980, 110, 131-35.

67. Krauss, R.M., Wood, P.D., Giotas, C., Waterman, D., and Lindgren, F.T. Circulation 1979, 60(Suppl. II):II-73.

68. Marniemi, J. and Hietanen, E. "Regulation of Serum Lipids by Physical Exercise"; CRC Press, 1982; pp. 116-8.

69. Simonelli, C. and Eaton, R.P. Ann. J. Physiol. 1978, 234, E221-7.
70. Dall'Aglio, E., Chang, F., Chang, H., Stern, J., and Reaven, G. Diabetes 1983, 32, 46-50.
71. Mela, D.J. and Kris-Etherton, P.M. Metabolism 1984, 33, 916-21.
72. Seelbach, J.D. and Kris-Etherton, P.M. Atherosclerosis, In press.
73. Gollnick, P.D. and Simmons, S.W. Int. Z. Angew. Physiol. 1967, 23, 322-30.
74. Gollnick, P.D. and Taylor, A.W. Int. Z. Angew. Physiol. 1969, 27, 144-53.
75. Robinson, L.A., Monsen, E.R., and Childs, M.T. Europ. J. Appl. Physiol. 1974, 33, 1-12.
76. Fukuda, N., Ide, T., Kida, Y., Takamine, K., and Sugano, M. Nutr. Metab. 1979, 23, 256-65.
77. Hebbklinck, M. and Casier, H. Int. Z. Angew. Physiol. 1969, 22, 185-9.
78. Simko, V. and Kelley, R.E. Atherosclerosis 1979, 32, 423-44.
79. Kramsch, D.M., Aspen, A.J., Abramowitz, B., Kreimendahl, T., and Hood, W., Jr. N. Eng. J. Med. 1981, 305, 1483-9.
80. Hasler, C., Rothenbacher, H., Mela, D., and Kris-Etherton, P.M. Atherosclerosis 1984, 52, 279-86.
81. Link, R.P., Pederosoli, W.M., and Safanie, A.H. Atherosclerosis 1972, 15, 107-22.
82. Wolffe, J.B., Digilio, V.A., Dale, A.D., McGinnis, G.E., Donnelly, D.J., Plungian, M.B., Sprowls, J., James, F., Einhorn, C., and Werkheiser, G. Am. Heart J. 1949, 38, 467. Abstract.
83. Wolffe, J.B., Hyman, A.S., Plungian, M.B., Dale, A.D., McGinnis, G.F., and Walkow, M.B. J. Gerontol. 1952, 7, 13-23.
84. Myasnikov, A.L. Circulation 1958, 17, 99-113.
85. Kobernick, S.D. and Niwayama, G. Am. J. Pathol. 1960, 36, 393-409.
86. Kobernick, S.D. and Hashimoto, T. Lab. Invest. 1963, 12, 638-47.
87. Prior, J.T. and Ziegler, D.D. Arch. Pathol. 1965, 80, 50-7.

RECEIVED June 10, 1985

6

Riboflavin Requirements and Exercise

Daphne A. Roe and Amy Z. Belko

Division of Nutritional Sciences, Savage Hall, Cornell University, Ithaca, NY 14853

Current questions frequently posed to nutritionists are whether people who are exercising have special vitamin needs and whether, if they have special needs, these can be met by a normal diet or whether they require nutrient supplements. A response to such questions can now be made with respect to a particular B vitamin, riboflavin.

Riboflavin deficiency and the dietary means to prevent such deficiency have been known since the late 1930's when early accounts of the clinical signs of riboflavin deficiency were published (1).

Clinical signs of riboflavin deficiency include fissures at the corners of the lips (angular stomatitis), dermatitis of skin creases, folds and areas of trauma (seborrhoeic dermatitis of the nasolabial folds, the periorbital creases and the inguinal areas, the vulva, and the scrotum), as well as peeling and/or fissuring of the lips (cheilosis) and sore tongue (glossitis). Other signs which are sometimes present include vascularization of the cornea, keratitis, blepharitis and anemia.

Subsequently, the functions of the vitamin were better established and requirements for the vitamin were set. Riboflavin is an integral part of two coenzymes, flavin-5'-phosphate (FMN) and flavin adenine dinucleotide (FAD), which function in oxidation/reduction reactions. Indeed, riboflavin is an enzyme cofactor which is necessary in metabolic processes in which oxidation of glucose or fatty acid is used for production of adenosine triphosphate (ATP) as well as in reactions in which oxidation of amino acids is accomplished. The minimum requirement for riboflavin has been established as that amount which actually prevents the signs of deficiency. A range of intakes varying from 0.55 to 0.75 mg/day of riboflavin has been established as the minimum amount which is required to prevent appearance of deficiency signs.

Today, biochemical deficiency of riboflavin is accepted in the absence of clinical signs of deficiency. Biochemical signs of deficiency include change in the amount of the vitamin which is excreted in the urine, or change in the level of activity of a red blood cell (erythrocyte) enzyme, which is known as the erythrocyte glutathione reductase. Requirements for the vitamin are defined as that amount which will prevent both clinical and biochemical signs of deficiency.

0097-6156/86/0294-0080$06.00/0

How Have Optimum Intakes for Riboflavin Been Determined?

Whereas riboflavin functions as a coenzyme of flavoproteins, which
are concerned with biological oxidations or energy utilization, it
has been proposed that with increased energy expenditure, the body's
need for riboflavin may be increased. In the past, the assessment of
riboflavin nutriture was primarily dependent on measurement of the
urinary excretion of the vitamin. If riboflavin intake is low,
excretion of the vitamin is diminished. As riboflavin intake is
increased to meet need, riboflavin excretion in the urine increases.
Indeed, urinary excretion of riboflavin both by adults and children
on diets containing up to approximately 0.5 mg riboflavin/1000 Kcal
is low and the excretion rises sharply as the dietary intake is
increased to 0.75 mg/1000 Kcal or above (2). Since 1972 red cell
enzyme assay of riboflavin status has been widely used.   Indeed, in
epidemiological and clinical studies of riboflavin status, the erythrocyte (red cell) glutathione reductase assay (EGR) is the test
which is usually undertaken. In 1972 Tillotson and Baker (3) showed
that this enzyme assay was sensitive to riboflavin depletion. It has
further been shown that change in this red cell enzyme activity is
one of the first changes to be found with reduction in intake of the
vitamin below need (4,5). Arguments have been published in favor of
relating standards for riboflavin requirements to food-energy intake
(6,7). However, since in the past no satisfactory evidence was
obtained from studies of the urinary excretion of riboflavin that
riboflavin requirements were increased when energy utilization was
increased, allowances for this vitamin in the United States have been
set for people engaging in "normal" activity (i.e., neither sedentary
nor engaged in heavy physical work) (8), and no modification of
intake has been recommended, based on change in food-energy requirements.
     The current Recommended Dietary Allowance (RDA) for riboflavin
for young adult males and for nonpregnant, nonlactating young adult
women is set in the U.S. at the level of 0.6 mg/1000 Kcal(9).Inter-
nationally, recommendations for daily intakes of riboflavin vary.
Thus, in the Philippines which have the lowest recommended dietary
intake for riboflavin, the level is set at 0.5 mg/1000 Kcal, while in
the USSR it is set at 0.79 mg/1000 Kcal. In several countries including Bulgaria, Chili, The People's Republic of China, Czechoslovakia,
Hungary, India, The Netherlands, Poland, Taiwan and the USSR, the
recommended dietary intakes for riboflavin vary with occupational or
energy expenditure categories (10).

Is There Experimental Evidence That Riboflavin Requirements Are
Influenced by the Level of Physical Activity?

Tucker et al. showed that both sudden severe physical exercise and
longer sustained work on a treadmill during training decreases urinary riboflavin excretion during the experimental periods (11). The
acute reduction in riboflavin excretion observed by these investigators was attributed to a reduction in renal plasma flow. In order to
explain the long-term reduced excretion of the vitamin, they proposed
that riboflavin was retained for incorporation into "new muscle
tissue". The significance of this study is that if the hypotheses

put forward were proven, it would mean that riboflavin requirements are increased with exercise, but in relation to change in lean body mass rather than due to change in energy expenditure.

In a 1979 study we showed that female volunteers who were fed diets for 10 weeks with either ascending or descending riboflavin content required intakes equal to or greater than 0.7 mg/riboflavin/1000 Kcal in order to normalize their EGR values. In a second study carried out by us which was designed to examine the effects of oral contraceptives on riboflavin requirements, 18 female subjects were fed ascending levels of dietary riboflavin until EGR values were normalized. No significant group differences were found between pill users and non-pill users in the amounts of riboflavin required to normalize the EGR. However, it was found that those subjects with the highest food-energy requirements also had high requirements for riboflavin. The subjects with the highest riboflavin requirements were also those who performed the greatest amount of physical activity (12-14).

We then carried out a further study in which the effects of exercise on riboflavin requirements of young women of normal body weight were assessed (15). During a 12 week study, subjects followed a six-week, sedentary period by a six-week exercise period in which they jogged around a track for 20 or 50 minutes per day. The study participants were aged 19-27 years. They were fed a basic diet containing 0.6 mg riboflavin/1000 Kcal of food intake. Their riboflavin intake in a diet of defined calorie content was increased by 0.2 mg/1000 Kcal increments by provision of riboflavin in a glucose polymer mixture. Linear regression analysis was used to estimate the riboflavin intake required for an EGR activity coefficient of 1.25 during both the no exercise and exercise period. Individual riboflavin requirements ranged from 0.62 to 1.21 mg/1000 Kcal before exercise. The riboflavin requirement for an EGR activity coefficient of <1.25 was increased from 0.96 mg/1000 Kcal during the nonexercise period to 1.1 mg/1000 Kcal during exercise. (Mean requirements B_2/1000 Kcal $\pm$ S.D. Pre-exercise period = 0.92 $\pm$ 0.17; Mean requirements B_2/1000 Kcal $\pm$ S.D. Exercise period = 1.12 $\pm$ 0.21.) Findings of this study led us to conclude that young, healthy women require more riboflavin to achieve biochemical normality than the 1980 RDA and that exercise increases their riboflavin requirements.

In a further study, we examined the effects of aerobic exercise and weight loss on the riboflavin requirements of moderately obese young women. The experiment was designed as a two period cross-over study with an initial baseline period and two 5-week metabolic periods. The basic diet of the subjects contained 1200 Kcal with a riboflavin concentration of 0.8 mg/1000 Kcal. Exercise in this study consisted of a program of aerobic dance. Riboflavin depletion as measured by increased EGR activity coefficients and decreased urinary excretion of riboflavin occurred during both non-exercise and exercise periods. The EGR activity coefficients increased from a baseline mean of 1.28 $\pm$ 0.11 to 1.40 $\pm$ 0.12 during non-exercise, and to 1.49 $\pm$ 0.16 during exercise. The urinary excretion of riboflavin fell during non-exercise and then further during the exercise period. The riboflavin depletion of these subjects was not correlated to the rate of weight loss which occurred during the study, nor to the composition of weight loss, nor to changes in their aerobic capacity (16).

As indicated above, in our studies of young women of normal weight, we estimated that while relatively sedentary they require in the order of 0.96 mg riboflavin/1000 Kcal of food-energy intake per day. During exercise periods they need in the order of 1.16 mg riboflavin/1000 Kcal/day.

In a further study of weight reducing women, we again found that riboflavin requirements for women who are exercising are on the average about 1.16 mg/1000 Kcal or greater (17).

Does Riboflavin Supplementation Improve Aerobic Capacity or Exercise Performance?

In our studies of young women whose intakes of riboflavin were at physiological levels, we did not find that the riboflavin intake above the RDA improved maximum aerobic capacity (17).

In a study carried out in Canada the effects of riboflavin supplementation on the nutritional status and athletic performance of elite swimmers was investigated (18). Fourteen swimmers including 8 men and 6 women participated in the study. They were divided into two groups on the basis of sex and performance level, such that each group comprised 4 men and 3 women. One group was given a 60 mg/day riboflavin supplement for 16-20 days. Both groups ingested a diet which met or exceeded Canadian recommended dietary allowances. Two tests were used to evaluate performance of the subjects. They submitted to a swimming test consisting of six 50 minute meter freestyle lengths, each separated by a ten second interval; the total time of the six lengths was used as an index of athletic performance. The second test was a stepwise incremental exercise to exhaustion performed on a treadmill. All subjects had normal riboflavin status before the experiment. The supplementation did not change EGR activity in the subjects. Riboflavin supplements had no influence on swimming performance and no relationship was found between EGR activity and VO_{2max} (18).

Examination of the literature has revealed that only one investigator has obtained evidence that riboflavin supplementation alters muscular activity (19). Haralambie studied a group of athletes before and after administration of 10 mg riboflavin. He found that there was a moderate change in neuromuscular irritability of specific muscle groups in the legs during electrical stimulation of the muscles, which was attributed to the treatment.

Can the Riboflavin Requirements of Athletes be Met by Food Sources of Riboflavin?

We are of the opinion that at least in young women such as those we have studied, riboflavin requirements of females who are undertaking aerobic exercise can be met by normal food sources of riboflavin. Rich food sources of riboflavin in the U.S. diet include milk, cheese, yogurt, fortified breakfast cereals, and to a lesser extent, enriched bread. The riboflavin content of commonly consumed foods is shown in Table I. We assume, however, that it might be difficult for exercisers to meet their riboflavin requirements if for one reason or another they were unable to consume milk or other dairy products.

For these people, it might be necessary to add a dietary supplement of riboflavin. In our own studies we have no specific experience of the riboflavin needs of men who are undertaking aerobic exercise, nor have we examined the riboflavin needs of those who undertake endurance tests.

Table I: Riboflavin Content of Popular Foods

Food/Beverage	Riboflavin mg
Whole milk (8 oz.)	0.41
Skim milk (8 oz.)	0.44
Cheeseburger (McDonalds) (1)	0.23
Beef and cheese sandwich (Arby's)	0.43
Chili (Wendy's)	0.25
Beef burrito (Taco Bell)	0.39
Whole wheat bread (1 slice)	0.06
Cornflakes (3/4 cup)	0.26
Cottage cheese (1/2 cup)	0.26
Chocolate pudding (1/2 cup)	0.18

In conclusion, we have found that the presently set Recommended Dietary Allowances for riboflavin for women are inadequate even when they are not exercising, and that their riboflavin requirements are increased by exercise. Weight reduction per se does not have an effect on riboflavin requirements. However, women who are exercising and on a weight reduction diet may get an inadequate amount of the vitamin because of their restricted food intake. We have no evidence, at least in the U.S., that athletes are at risk for clinical riboflavin deficiency. We do not think that it is necessary for those engaged in exercise to take megadoses of this B vitamin or of other B vitamins.

Summary

Riboflavin requirements can be defined as that amount of the vitamin, also called vitamin B_2, which will prevent both clinical and biochemical signs of deficiency. The current Recommended Dietary Allowance for riboflavin is set at 0.6 mg for every 1000 Kilocalories of food-energy consumed per day. This is the amount of the vitamin which, in the opinion of the Food and Nutrition Board of the National Research Council (National Academy of Sciences) will meet the needs of most healthy people. Recent studies, however, have shown that healthy young women require more riboflavin than this when they are sedentary and that their requirements for the vitamin increase when they exercise. The increased needs of healthy women for riboflavin can be met if women increase their intake of rich food sources of the vitamin including milk, cheese, and yogurt. No special athletic advantage is to be gained by taking megadoses of riboflavin.

Literature Cited

1. Sebrell, W. H. & Butler, R. E. (1939) Riboflavin deficiency in man. Public Health Reports 54, 2121-31.
2. Horwitt, M. K., Harvey, C. C., Hills, O. W. & Liebert, E. (1950) Correlation of urinary excretion of riboflavin with dietary intake and symptoms of ariboflavinosis. J. Nutr. 41, 247-64.
3. Tillotson, J. A. & Baker, E. M. (1972) An enzymatic measurement of the riboflavin status in man. Am. J. Clin. Nutr. 25, 425-431.
4. Sauberlich, H. E. Judd, J. H. Nichoalds, G. E. Broquist, H.P. & Darby, W. J. (1972) Application of the erythrocyte glutathione reductase assay in evaluating riboflavin nutritional status in a high school student population. Am. J. Clin. Nutr. 25, 756-62.
5. Thurnham, D. I. (1981) Red cell enzyme tests of vitamin status: do marginal deficiencies have any physiological significance? Proc. Nutr. Soc. 40, 155-62.
6. Bro-Rasmussen, F. (1958) The riboflavin requirements of animals and man and associated metabolic relations. Nutr. Abst. Rev. 28, 1-23.
7. Bro-Rasmussen, F. (1958) The riboflavin requirement of animals and man and associated metabolic relations. II. Relation of requirement to the metabolism of protein and energy. Nutr. Abst. Rev. 28, 369-86.
8. Horwitt, M. K. (1966) Nutritional requirements of man with special reference to riboflavin. Am. J. Clin. Nutr. 18, 458-66.
9. "Recommended Dietary Allowances", 8th and 9th Rev. Ed. (1974, 1980) Washington, D.C. Food and Nutrition Board, National Academy of Sciences.
10. "Recommended Dietary Intakes Around the World". A report by Committee 1/5 of the International Union of Nutritional Sciences (1983). Part I. Nutr. Abst. Rev. 53, 939-1015.
11. Tucker, R. G. Mickelsen, O. & Keys, A. (1960) The infuence of sleep, work, diuresis, acute starvation, thiamine intake, and bed rest on human riboflavin excretion. J. Nutr. 72, 251-61.
12. Roe, D. A., Mueller, K. & Bogusz, S. (1980) Riboflavin requirements of young women. Fed. Proc. 39, 552.
13. Roe, D.A. (1981) Intergroup and intragroup variables affecting interpretation of studies of drug effects on nutritional status. In: "Nutrition in Health and Disease In International Development"; XII Internat. Congr. Nutr. Sympo., New York: Alan R. Liss, Inc., p. 767-771.
14. Roe, D. A., Bogusz, S., Sheu, J. & McCormick, D. B. (1982) Factors affecting riboflavin requirements of oral contraceptive users and non-users. Am. J. Clin. Nutr. 35, 495-501.
15. Belko, A. Z., Obarzanek, E., Kalkwarf, H. J., Rotter, M. A., Bogusz, S., Miller, D., Haas, J. D. & Roe, D. A. (1983) Effects of exercise on riboflavin requirements of young women. Am. J. Clin. Nutr. 37, 509-17.
16. Belko, A. Z., Obarzanek, E., Roach, R., Rotter, M., Urban, G., Weinberg, S. & Roe, D.A. (1984) Effects of aerobic exercise and weight loss on riboflavin requirements of moderately obese,

marginally deficient young women.   Am.   J.   Clin.   Nutr. $\underline{40}$,   553-61.

17.   Belko,   A.   Z.,   Meredith,   M.   P.,   Kalkwarf,   H.   J.,   Obarzanek,   E.,   Weinberg,   S.,   Roach,   R.,   McKeon,   G.   &   Roe,   D.   A.   (1985)   Effects of exercise on riboflavin requirements: biological validation in weight reducing women.   Am.   J.   Clin.   Nutr. $\underline{41}$,   270-77.

18.   Tremblay,   A.,   Boilard,   F.,   Breton,   M-F.,   Bessette, $\overline{\text{H}}$.   &   Roberge,   A.   G.   (1984)   The effects of riboflavin supplementation on the the nutritional status and performance of elite swimmers.   Nutr.   Res. $\underline{4}$,   201-8.

19.   Haralambie,   G.   (1976)   Vitamin B_2 status in athletes and the influence   of riboflavin administration on   neuromuscular   irritablity.   Nutr.   Metabol. $\underline{20}$,   1-8.

RECEIVED May 30, 1985

Trace Elements and Calcium Status in Athletic Activity

Roger McDonald[1] and Paul Saltman[2]

[1] The Department of Physical Education, University of Southern California, Los Angeles, CA 90089
[2] The Department of Biology, University of California at San Diego, La Jolla, CA 92093

Throughout the centuries the athlete has embraced special foods and diets as a means of providing the "winning edge". The years of trial and error to establish the effect of nutrition on performance have resulted in a plethora of myths which engulf the area of nutrition and sport. This may partially explain the differences that exist in in our perceptions and definitions of the study of nutrition. To the scientist, nutrition is the elucidation of the nutrients required to permit optimal growth, development and performance of the individual. Little attention is paid to the psychology, anthropology and sociology of food. Conversely, the general population, and the athletes in particular, believe that food and diets are equivalent to nutrition. The psychology, or more appropriately the metaphysics, of food plays a significant role in nutrition. The athlete may determine his/her diet based largely on social, ethnic, and economic issues rather than on the nutrient value. This review will be concerned primarily with the biochemistry and physiology of nutrition. However, the reader should not disregard the myths of the training table as a principal determinant in the nutrition of the athlete.

The ability to perform even the simplest of muscle movement requires complex coordination of the physical and chemical activities of the tissue. In recent years, nutritionists and exercise physiologists have described how the primary energy sources in food carbohydrates, fats, and proteins are transformed into the universal "currency" of biological energy, ATP. Oxidative metabolism processes the substrates through a cascade of enzymatic events to insure maximal efficiency in energy conversion. At every level of this conversion, one or more metal ions serve as a cofactor to facilitate these biochemical reactions. The requirement of metals in the production of

0097–6156/86/0294–0087$06.00/0

energy is evident. However, with the exception of iron, there exists
a paucity of definitive studies describing the affects of other trace
metals on physical performance. We will focus our initial attention
on iron, then explore the role of calcium and its participation in
exercise. Finally we will relate the other trace element requirements to physical activity.

Iron

Biological Role of Iron. The vast majority of iron within the body
directly participates in the transportation and metabolic utilization of oxygen. Some iron is involved in the redox reactions of metabolism. The rest is stored. Table I presents a partial list of
iron-containing proteins. The normal human adult contains approximately 2.5 g of iron (1). Of this, 70% exists within the red blood
cells as hemoglobin. The storage protein ferritin, which acts as a
mobilizable reserve of iron, accounts for another 25% of total body
iron. The remaining 5% exists within the tissues as myoglobin, enzymes, or transferrin.
        Myoglobin contains a significant fraction of the iron in muscle
tissue. Once thought to function only as an oxygen storage protein,
recent evidence suggests that myoglobin acts primarily to facilitate
oxygen diffusion between the capillary and tissue membrane (2).
Other iron-containing enzymes play an integral role in oxidative
respiration such as mitochondrial cytochromes, catalase, peroxidase
and other heme iron proteins. The non-heme iron-sulfur proteins,
NADH-dehydrogenase, succinate dehydrogenase and xanthine oxidase account for the largest portion of iron within the mitochondria. The
glycolytic and mitochondrial enzyme, alpha-glycerolphosphate dehydrogenase, also contains an iron atom in an unknown form.

Nutritional Considerations. Dietary iron deficiency ranks second to
obesity among the major nutritional problems in the United States.
Nutritional surveys have indicated that as many as 57% of the total
American population and 90% of the women do not obtain the recommended dietary allowance (10 mg/day for men and 18 mg/day for women)
(3, 4). Nutritional iron deficiency among infants and the young is
common and most prevalent in lower socioeconomic groups (5). Studies
describing nutritional iron deficiency among athletes have been slow
in forthcoming. However, a recent study completed in our laboratory
suggests that highly trained endurance athletes do not ingest the
RDA for iron (6). Some authors have suggested that athletes suffer
'sports anemia', an anemia associated with exercise (7). It has been
difficult to ascertain either the extent or etiology of this condition.
        The diagnosis of iron deficiency has its difficulties and ambi-
guities. Severe iron deficiency can be detected easily by the marked
reduction in hemoglobin concentration, mean corpuscular hemoglobin
and decreased serum iron concentration. However, in mild iron deficiency hemoglobin concentration, transferrin saturation, and serum
ferritin levels are frequently normal in patients with depleted bone

Table I   Representative Iron Proteins

Protein	Iron Form	Location	Function
Hemoglobin	Heme	Erythrocytes	Oxygen transport
Myoglobin	Heme	Cytosol	Facilitation of oxygen diffusion
Cytochromes	Heme	Mitochondria	Electron transport
Succinate dehydrogenase	Iron-Sulfur	Mitochondria	Reduction of succinate to fumate
NADH-dehydrogenase	Iron-Sulfur	Cytosol/Mitochondria	Oxidation of NADH to NAD^+
Catalase	Heme	Peroxisomes	$H_2O_2 \rightarrow H_2O + \frac{1}{2}O_2$
Xanthing oxidase	Iron-Sulfur	Cytosol	Oxidation of xanthine to uric acid
Alpha-glycerolphosphate dehydrogenase	?	Cytosol/Mitochondria	Shuttle for reducing equivalents
Aconitase	Iron-Sulfur	Mitochondria	Isomerase in Krebs cycle
Monamine oxidase	?	Mitochondria	Control of neurotransmitters

marrow iron stores (8,9). The uncertainty of detecting iron deficiency was recently pointed out by Rivera et al. (10). These investigators supplemented apparently normal Mexican school children
(Hb = 13.5 - 14.0 g/dl) with iron fortified milk. Supplementation
increased hemoglobin concentration by 10% in the entire population
within 10 weeks. This was a surprising finding since others have
suggested that hemoglobin concentration in normal groups does not
respond to iron supplementation. Hemoglobin concentration, alone,
can be a poor indicator of iron status.

Iron and Work Performance. There is a direct correlation of iron deficiency with impaired physical work performance. As early as 1942,
Karpovick and Millman (11) reported declining performance of athletes
due to a reduction of hemoglobin concentration following blood dona-
tion. Other early descriptive investigations confirmed these data
(12, 13). However, it was not until the late 1950's that Beutler et
al. (14) were able to objectively establish a correlation between
hemoglobin concentration and total body oxygen consumption, considered to be the best measure of work performance capacity. Hemoglobin
concentration increased at the same rate as oxygen consumption during
a submaximal work performance task following three weeks of iron supplementation of anemic subjects. Additional support for these data
has been accumulated by Gardner et al. (15) and Edgerton et al. (16)
in an anemic population of female Sri Lankan tea farm workers. Gardner et al. (15) described the work performance changes in a brief
intense type of exercise. Mild anemia resulted in decreased work
performance, as measured by maximal oxygen consumption (15). The
close relation between maximal work times and hemoglobin concentration found in these women is seen in Figure 1. Edgerton et al. (16)
measured extended submaximal work capacity. Following three weeks of
iron supplementation, activity levels and tea picking production were
increased by as much as 60% over the control group or placebo treatment. This increase was correlated directly with an elevation in
hemoglobin concentrations.

The Sri Lankan investigations could be questioned because the
population may have suffered from other nutritional deficiencies as
well. The question must then be asked "Would low hemoglobin concentrations affect performance in otherwise healthy, well nourished individuals?" Ekblom et al. (17) studied the work performance capacity
of healthy physical education students both before and after removal
of 800 ml or 1200 ml of blood. Oxygen consumption decreased by 13%
and 18% in the two groups, respectively. Woodson and coworkers (18)
suggested that a decrease in work performance due to blood removal
could not be explained by a decrease in blood volume. Replacement
of whole blood with equal volumes of isotonic saline did not restore
work performance in rats. Thus, hemoglobin concentration appears to
be a singular rate-limiting factor in work performance.

If decreased hemoglobin concentration results in impaired work
performance, what effect would an increase in hemoglobin have on exercise? This question has been answered by reinfusing packed erythrocytes into endurance athletes, a procedure known as blood doping.

Buick et al. (19) used a double-blind experiment in which either
packed erythrocytes or saline solutions were infused into highly
trained endurance runners. Their results indicated that an increase
in hematocrit produces significantly greater work capacity when compared to sham control or pre-infusion values. While these findings
have been supported by others (20), Murray et al. (21) cautioned
against increasing the hematocrit level above 50% (pcv). At elevated
hematocrits, work performance fell as a result of increased viscosity
of the blood.

Iron deficiency can lead to a decrease in tissue iron proteins
and enzymes. The loss of metabolic activity of the respiratory iron
enzymes may result in a decrease in physical work performance (24,
25). Using iron-deficient rats, these investigators adjusted hemoglobin concentration to normal levels with blood transfusions without
affecting the tissue iron stores. After the anemia was corrected by
the transfusion, decreased work performance was still observed. They
attributed impaired work performance to low levels of alpha-glycerolphosphate dehydrogenase- and iron-containing glycolytic enzyme. This
finding was surprising since the contribution of this enzyme to the
total energy production in the mammal is relatively small (26). Other
investigators have failed to confirm the results of Finch (27, 29).

Iron-containing muscle proteins, such as myoglobin, cytochrome
c, and succinate dehydrogenase, play a critical role in mammalian oxidative respiration and could well be rate-limiting during work performance (29-31). Davies et al. (29) studied the maximal work performance and endurance capacity of iron-deficient rats during seven
days of iron repletion. Hemoglobin concentration increased in paral-
lel with maximal work performance (Figure 2). However, endurance
capacity did not increase until the mitochondrial enzymes pyruvate
kinase, cytochrome c and NADH dehydrogenase showed significant increases over control animals. The alpha glycerolphosphate shuttle
system was reported not to contribute significantly to either type
of work performance.

The ability of iron deficiency to disrupt physical work performance by affecting both oxygen transport and oxidative energy metabolism makes iron-deficient animals an ideal model for studying cellular energy capacity. This approach was taken by McDonald et al. (30)
in a study to characterize changes in the myoglobin concentration of
control- and iron-deficient exercising rats. Iron-deficient animals,
when subjected to an exercise regime, can gradually increase their
submaximal work performance to levels attained by iron-normal animals
(Figure 3). This increase could be directly correlated with increased
myoglobin concentration, without any change in hemoglobin values.
However, when the anemic animal is worked beyond submaximal effort,
the oxygen content of the blood may fall below requirements needed
to sustain exercise (Figure 4). These results confirmed the hypothesis of Davies et al. (29) that oxygen carrying capacity (hemoglobin)
limits intense exercise and cellular oxidative energy metabolism regulates extended mild exercise.

Calcium

Biological Role of Calcium. Calcium represents a large weight fraction of the elemental composition of the human body. Of the 1.3 kg of

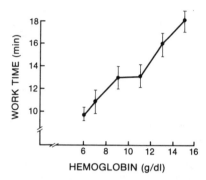

Figure 1. Maximal treadmill work time and hemoglobin concentration of Sri Lanken women. Data from Ref. 15.

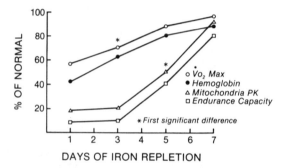

Figure 2. Hemoglobin, Maximal oxygen consumption (VO₂ max), mitochondrial pyruvate kinase (PK), and endurance capacity of rats during seven days of iron repletion. Data from Ref. 29.

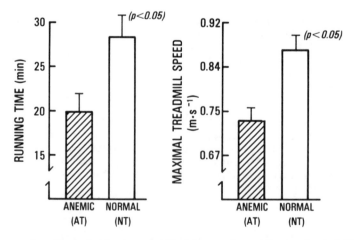

Figure 3. Mean daily treadmill times of anemic trained (AT) and normal trained (NT) rats. Reproduced with permission from Ref. 30. Copyright 1984 Springer-Verlag New York, Inc.

calcium distributed throughout the body, approximately 99% exists within the bones (32, 33). The other 1% (15g) is distributed in teeth (7g), soft tissue (7g), plasma (300 mg), and extravascular fluid (700 mg). Because of the large calcium content of bone, the description of the biological role of calcium necessitates a discussion of bone metabolism. However, it is not the purpose of this paper to provide an exhaustive review of bone physiology. The following sections will discuss the importance of calcium in bone and as a metabolic participant in exercise. Reviews detailing bone physiology have been written by Glimcher (33), Urist (34), Heaney (35) and Vaughan (36).

Calcium performs a variety of cellular functions in muscle and nerve that ultimately result in muscular contraction. Excellent descriptions of calcium's function in muscle and nerve are to be found in the reviews by Hoyle (37), Cohen (38), and Robertson (39). At the neuromuscular junction, the excitable cells are very sensitive to changes in extracellular concentrations of calcium. Curtis (40) and Luttgau (41) described a fall in the resting action potential and electrical resistance when the extracellular calcium concentration fell below 10^{-4} M. The action potential and electrical resistance returned to normal following addition of calcium to this *in vitro* preparation. The magnitude of the initial muscle membrane action potential, that which regulates the propagation of further muscle contraction, is also mediated by the extracellular calcium concentration. While the inward flow of sodium ions from the extracellular space remains the dominant factor in the mechanism of muscle membrane depolarization, calcium ion flux appears to mediate the cell's permeability to sodium ions. This effect is particularly true in cardiac tissue (42).

Heibrunn and Wiercinsk (43) were the first to describe the importance of calcium to muscular contraction. Their findings were later applied to Huxley's element theory of muscular contraction (44, 45) by Hoyle (46) and Cohen (38). As the contraction propagates throughout the muscle fiber, the depolarization descends the transverse tubules (T-tubules) within the sarcoplasmic reticulum where calcium is released in proximity to the contractile proteins. The intracellular concentration of calcium rises rapidly from a resting state of 10^{-8} M to 10^{-5} M. The calcium then binds to a specific site on the troponin protein affixed to the actin filament. While the precise mechanism of action on the actin filament is unclear, it appears that calcium stimulates a structural rotation of the troponin-tropomyosin complex. The rotation of the actin filament exposes the tropomyosin to the myosin cross-bridge which allows binding of actin and myosin required for contraction. When the depolarization stimulus is withdrawn, calcium is sequestered and relaxation of the muscle ensues. It also should be noted that the supply of glucose to the working muscle from glycogen appears to be mediated by calcium-stimulated activation of phosphorylase (47). The conversion of inactive phosphorylase b to active phosphorylase a occurs at a calcium concentration equal to that needed for mechanical contraction.

Calcium ions also regulate nerve cell permeability to sodium and potassium, and in turn affect nerve transmission (48). Further, calcium enhances the release of acetylcholine at the neuromuscular junctions (49). Figure 5 presents a schematic summary of the events

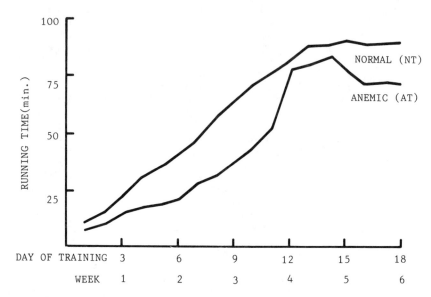

Figure 4. Maximal run times and maximal treadmill speed of anemic
trained (AT) and normal trained (NT) rats following six weeks of
endurance training.   Reproduced with permission from Ref. 30.
Copyright 1984 Springer- Verlag New York, Inc.

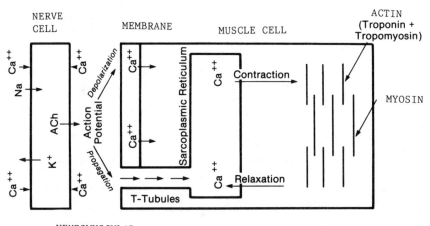

Figure 5. Schematic summary of calcium's role in muscle contraction.

occuring in the muscle and nerve in which calcium affects muscle contraction.

Calcium Requirements. Calcium and its richest dietary source, milk,
has frequently been regarded as a nutrient only for the young.
However, the need for calcium throughout the life cycle is fundamental. Calcium intake must be sufficient to maintain positive calcium balance at all times. However, conflicting results from numerous investigations have raised questions concerning the adequacy of
the current U.S. RDA of 800 mg of calcium per day. The normal adult
body requires an average of 500-600 mg of calcium per day in order to
maintain positive calcium balance. Young adults have been reported
to remain in positive balance at intakes of calcium as low as 420 mg/
day (50). On the other hand, postmenopausal women were found to be
in negative calcium balance with intakes of 800 mg/day. The decrease
in intestinal absorption of calcium that occurs naturally with aging
may also affect calcium balance. Calcium requirements among the
elderly are difficult to ascertain due to the influence of decreased
physical activity, possible vitamin D deficiency, and loss of hormone
production. Further, the intake of dietary protein, phosphorus, carbohydrate, and fats can directly or indirectly influence calcium balance (51-54).

Studies by Nordin et al. (32), Albanese et al. (55) and Smith
et al. (56) have suggested increasing dietary calcium for the elderly
and postmenopausal women in order to prevent bone mineral loss and
the concomitant increased risk of osteoporosis. The importance of
calcium supplementation in preventing bone loss has not gone without
question. Garn et al. (57) studied 13,000 subjects from seven different countries and was unable to find any relationship between calcium intake and the incidence of osteoporosis in either sex. These
investigators concluded that bone loss is a general phenomenon of
aging in humans and that factors other than calcium intake play a
more significant role in the development of osteoporosis. Lack of
physical activity (58, 59), postmenopausal estrogen loss (55) and
altered bone metabolism (60) can all play a key role in the development of osteoporosis.

Calcium and Exercise. While there exists a widespread belief that
exercise can promote better health and prevent disease, little scientific data has been accumulated to support this contention. In the
case of prevention of bone mineral loss by physical activity, it is
clear that mineral loss in the elderly and increased bone density in
athletes is a distinct function of activity (56,61). These observations
have encouraged the use of exercise as a required modality in the
prevention and treatment of osteoporosis.

Albright (62) was the first to demonstrate that the lack of physical activity leads to a decrease in bone mineralization and the
development of osteoporosis. Subsequent studies supported these
findings and described the reversal of bone loss through exercise.
Smith (58) reported that physical activity among aged women (55-94
years) slowed the normal process of bone loss. Low intensity passive
physical therapy as well as simple weight-bearing movement increased
bone mineral content as much as 7.6% above a non-active control group
(Figure 6). Smith et al. (58) reported increases in bone mineral
content of aging females following three years of exercise. The

exercise group showed an increase of 2.3% in mineral content, while
the non-active control group declined by 3.3%.

Additional support for the role of exercise has been observed in
individuals subjected to the weightlessness of space (63). Astronauts
participating in Gemini IV, V, and VII orbital missions reported
small but significant bone mineral loss in flights lasting as few as
five days. However, the crew of Gemini VII, a space flight of 14
days, suffered the least bone loss because of an on-board isometric
and isotonic exercise program. Athletes also show an increase in
bone mineral content following exercise. World class athletes had
significantly more dense femoral bones than groups of inactive and
moderately active persons (61). Increased bone mineral content was
related to the athlete's specific sport. Weight lifters had greater
bone mineral content than throwers; throwers greater than runners;
runners greater than swimmers. The increase in bone mineral content
does not appear to be affected by age. Middle-aged (30-49 years)
marathon runners developed more dense femoral bones than did age-
matched controls (64).

Although most studies of bone density and exercise have been
performed on humans, a few investigators have described bone mineral
changes using animal models. Rats performing weight lifting (65) and
running exercise (66) developed both increased mineral mass and
breaking stress in femurs when compared with bones from sedentary
animals. Calcium content, measured directly in dry ashed bones, increased in all rats following exercise. Exercise also increases the
non-mineralized organic matrix in the bones (67, 68). Collagen formation, as measured by bone hydroxyproline, significantly increased in
adult rats following eight weeks of treadmill running.

Exercise and Urinary Calcium Excretion. Lack of physical acitivity
in prolonged bed-rest causes an increase in urinary calcium (69, 70).
Balance studies have shown that this hypercalciuria is not due to increased intestinal absorption of calcium (71). A reduction in dietary intake of calcium does not prevent calciuria (72). The cause
appears to be an imbalance between the rate of bone formation and
resorption which occurs after the loss of weight-bearing stress (73).
Issekutz et al. (70) reported that complete bed-rest for 42 days resulted in a doubling of urinary calcium excretion by male subjects.
Supine exercise up to four hours/day did not prevent the increase.
However, three hours/day of quiet standing proved to be sufficient to
induce a slow decline of the elevated calcium excretion. While it is
clear that the loss of gravitational stress causes elevated urinary
calcium, exercise may also create conditions which lead to increased
calciuria. In a recently completed study, McDonald (74) reported increased urinary calcium following prolonged exercise in both highly
trained endurance athletes and normal active controls (Figure 7).
Although absolute values for calcium excretion were higher in the
trained group following exercise, calcium excretion was 20-30% greater for both groups.

Increased urinary calcium following exercise may be caused by
the onset of metabolic acidosis associated with prolonged exercise.
Elevation of urinary calcium has been noted in studies where metabolic acidosis was induced by feeding an acid ash diet (75), hydro-
chloric acid (76), or ammonium chloride (77). Renal tubular acidosis can also induce elevated urinary calcium (78). Walser (79) re-

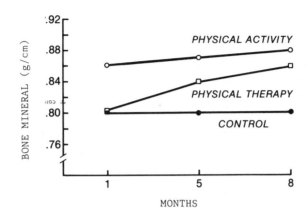

Figure 6.   Bone mineral content of elderly individuals following physical activity or physical therapy   Data from Ref. 56.

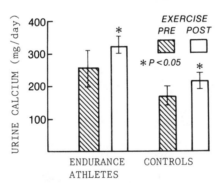

Figure 7.   Urinary calcium of highly trained and moderately active individuals before and after prolonged exercise.

ported that increased metabolic acidosis inhibited the proximal
tubular reabsorption of calcium, thus causing an increase in excretion. The effect of exercise-induced metabolic acidosis on urinary
calcium loss has not been investigated.

Copper and Zinc

Copper and zinc play important roles in a wide variety of biological
functions. However, their contribution to exercise performance has
yet to be evaluated directly. The participation of these elements in
muscle activity provides fruitful areas for further exercise physiology research. Detailed reviews of copper metabolism have been written by Underwood (80), O'Dell (81), and Li (82). Extensive reviews
of zinc metabolism have been provided by Prasad (83), Li (82), Underwood (84), and Sandstead (85).

Biological Roles of Zinc and Copper. Zinc and copper are essential
cofactors at the active site of a number of enzymes. Zinc is a component of more than 200 proteins and enzymes (Table II). Copper, similar to iron, participates both in redox reactions and as a proton doner
(Table III). The normal human adult body contains approximately 50-
100 mg of copper and 2.0 g of zinc. The vast majority of tissue copper is found in the liver, kidney, heart and brain. In the blood,
copper exists within the red blood cell as superoxide dismutase and
in the serum as ceruloplasmin. Copper is a component of aerobic
metabolism, bone synthesis, and erythrocyte development. Zinc is
found primarily in the liver, kidney, bone and prostate. Zinc is
essential for normal growth of tissues, wound repair, skin structure,
reproduction, taste perception, and the prevention of dwarfism.

Table II.   Representative Zinc Proteins

Protein	Location	Function
Carbonic anhydrase	Erythrocyte	$CO_2 + H_2O \leftrightarrow H_2CO_3$
DNA polymerase	Nucleus	DNA replication
RNA polymerase	Nucleus	RNA transcription
Alkaline phosphatase	Most tissues	Hydrolysis of phosphorous esters
Superoxide dismutase	Mitochondria	$2O_2^- + 2H^+ \rightarrow H_2O_2 + O_2$
Carboxypeptidase A & B	Pancreas	Hydrolysis of peptide bonds
Alcohol dehydrogenase	Liver	Oxidation of ethanol
Metallothionine	Most tissues	Zn and Cu storage

Table III.   Representative Copper Proteins

Protein	Location	Function
Ceruloplasmin	Serum	$Fe(II) \leftrightarrow Fe(III)+e^-$ Cu storage & transport
Dopamine beta-hydroxylase	Adrenal glands	Conversion of dopamine to norepinephrine
Cytochrome oxidase	Mitochondria	Terminal oxidase
Superoxide dismutase	Mitochondria	$2O_2^- + 2H^+ \rightarrow H_2O_2 + O_2$
Lysyl oxidase	Connective tissue	Formation of collagen cross-links
Tyrosinase	Skin	Pigmentation

Copper and Zinc in Aerobic Metabolism. Cytochrome oxidase, the terminal oxidase in the electron transport chain contains an atom of copper. On this enzyme the protons and electrons generated during oxidative metabolism combine with elemental oxygen to form water. During copper deficiency the tissue concentration of cytochrome oxidase is reduced. While the effects of lower cytochrome oxidase activity on exercise has not been described, it is likely that aerobic energy metabolism will be diminished. This effect of copper deficiency was first described in animals with myelin aplasis — the degeneration myelin (86). The oxidative process of phospholipid synthesis, a primary component of myelin, was depressed. Liver mitochondria had impaired respiratory activity (87). Cytochrome oxidase activity was also depressed in brain, heart and liver.

Superoxide dismutase, a copper- and zinc-containing mitochondrial enzyme, may play a significant role in exercise performance (88). Superoxide dismutase catalyzes the detoxification of oxygen-free radicals to oxygen and hydrogen peroxide. During exercise, it is proposed that the energy-yielding reactions of the mitochondria also produce potentially damaging superoxide. The rate of production of this compound is directly proportional to the rate of oxygen consumption. Since endurance training increases the total amount of mitochondria, the trained individual would have more dismutase and thus should be able to detoxify more superoxide. It would therefore appear that endurance training may decrease cellular damage caused by lipid membrane peroxidation. Since superoxide dismutase activity can be impaired by copper or zinc deficiency, the mechanism of this action should be experimentally explored.

Bone Disorders. Copper deficiency causes gross skeletal abnormalities in both humans and animal systems. Recently, our laboratory was able to induce experimental osteopenia in rats moderately deficient in copper and manganese (89). After one year on a low copper, low manganese diet, these animals showed reduced mineralization of calcium in femurs (Figure 8). The primary biochemical lesion in the

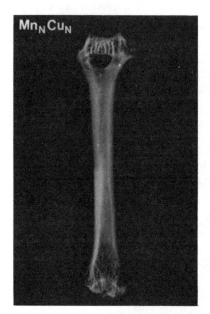

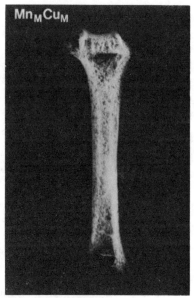

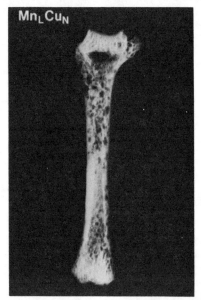

Figure 8. Radiographs of humeri from rats raised on either a con-
trol-normal ($Mn_n Cu_n$), or a moderate-manganese, moderate-copper
($Mn_m Cu_m$), or a manganese-free ($Mn_l Cu_n$) diet for 12 months.

bones of copper-deficient animals is a reduction in the activity of the copper enzyme lysyl oxidase, which plays a central role in the formation of cross-links in collagen and elastin (90). In a reaction that has not been fully elucidated, lysyl oxidase catalyzes the oxidative deamination of lysyl and hydroxylysyl residues. The resulting allysyl and hydroxyallysyl residues cross-link by spontaneously forming Schiff's bases. Calcification is reduced in the altered organic matrix.

Cardiovascular Disorders and Copper. Sudden cardiac failure has been associated with copper deficiency (91). There are two attractive mechanisms. First, the coronary arteries and aorta may become weakened from an inability to synthesize elastin due to a decrease in lysyl oxidase activity. Rupture of these major blood vessels has been shown to cause sudden death in animals suffering from copper deficiency. Second, a decrease in cytochrome oxidase activity during copper deficiency impairs aerobic metabolism of the heart and increases the risk of hypertrophy. Hypertrophy, which may lead to high output congestive heart failure, is exacerbated by hypochromic anemia also caused by copper deficiency.

Zinc and Immunity. Zinc is required for immunocompetence. Recently published reviews have detailed the role of zinc (92-95). Early clinical descriptions of zinc deficiency and impaired immune function were first reported by Brummerstedt et al.(96) who reported that calves with a genetically acquired inability to absorb zinc suffered from stunted growth, several skin disorders, viral and fungal infections, and atrophied thymus glands. These symptoms could be reversed by the administration of large amounts of dietary zinc.

The mechanism by which zinc mediates immune function is not clear; the depression of DNA synthesis during zinc deficiency is implicated (93). McDaffrey et al. (97) demonstrated that a zinc-containing DNA polymerase is present in the thymus but does not appear in the mature T cell. A reduction in thymus tissue caused by zinc deficiency would adversely affect the immunocompetence of thymocytes. This hypothesis has been confirmed in experiments where a sharp drop in the thymic hormone is induced by zinc deficiency.

While many a jogger has suggested that exercise can improve his/her resistance to infectious diseases, conclusive scientific evidence that exercise enhances immune response has yet to be presented. Experimental zinc deficiency in animals may provide a workable model for such investigations. It is well known that exercise induces hypertrophy of adrenal glands with a concomitant increase in the serum concentration of glucocorticoids. Zinc deficiency decreases T cell helper activity and thymic involution followed by a rise in glucocorticoids (98). The observations cited above suggest that it is possible to delineate experimentally the roles of zinc and exercise in immune response.

Summary

The essentiality of the trace elements and calcium for optimal physical performance is clear. The amount of dietary intake of these elements to achieve these levels is less clear. Our best estimates

are those given by the U.S. RDA's (Table IV). It is rather simple to
read and understand the dosage in those tables. But it is difficult
to be certain that the food intake does indeed supply the necessary
amounts. Most athletes who avail themselves of a wide variety of
foods including adequate meats and dairy products and who consume
calories sufficient to meet energy requirements, should be optimally
nourished. The need for supplemental trace elements is more in the
nature of "insurance" of athletic potency both physiologically and
psychologically. Certainly any regimen that suggests "mega-dosing"
of trace elements should be avoided. Every important trace element
and calcium is toxic at high concentrations. The body is not able
to adequately control uptake and storage of those vital nutrients at
excessive concentrations. Further, there is no reason to believe
that exercise increases the demand of the body for trace elements
much above that for the normal healthy non-competitive adult. In the
final analysis, the best friend of the athlete remains "good genes,
mental stamina, and disciplined training".

Table IV. Food and Nutrition Board, National Academy of Sciences-
           Recommended Daily Dietary Allowances for Adults

	Iron (mg)	Calcium* (mg)	Copper** (mg)	Zinc (mg)
Males	10	800	2	15
Females	18	800	2	15

*The National Academy is expected to increase this requirement to
 1000-1200 mg.

**This is a suggested amount. No official RDA has been established
 for copper.

Acknowledgments

We wish to thank Dr. Linda Strause for advice and counsel. This work
was supported in part by grants from the Weingart Foundation and
USPHS NIH Research Grant AM 12386.

Literature Cited

1. Hallberg, L. In "Present Knowledge in Nutrition, 5th Edition";
    The Nutrition Foundation, Washington D.C., 1984; p. 459.
2. Wittenberg, B. A.; Wittenberg, J. P.; Cadwell, P. J. Biol. Chem.
    1975, 250, 9038-43.
3. "Recommended Dietary Allowances"; National Academy of Sciences,
    1980, 9th ed.
4. "Ten State Nutrition Survey"; U. S. Dept. of HEW, 1972.
5. Karp, H.; Haaz, W.; Starko, K.; Gorman, J. M. Am. J. Dis. Child.
    1974, 128, 18-20.
6. McDonald, R. Unpublished data.
7. Yoshimura, H. Nutrition Reviews, 1970, 28, 252-3.
8. Beutler, E.; Drennan, W.; Block, M. J. Lab. Clin. Med. 1954,
    43, 427-39.

9. Hutchinson, K. <u>Blood</u> 1953, 8, 236–48.
10. Rivera, R.; Ruiz, R.; Hegenauer, J.; Saltman, P.; Green, R. Am. J. Clin. Nutr. 1982, 36, 1162–69.
11. Karpovich, P.; Millman, N. <u>Res. Quart. Am. Health Phys. Educ. Recr.</u> 1942, 166, 13–15.
12. Cullumbine, H. J. Appl. Physiol. 1949, 2, 274–77.
13. Kjellberg, S. R.; Ruhde, V.; Sjotrand, T. <u>Acta Physiol. Scand.</u> 1950, 19, 152–69.
14. Beutler, E.; Laush, S.; Tanzi, F. <u>Amer. J. Med. Sci.</u> 1960, 239, 759–65.
15. Gardner, G. W.; Edgerton, V. R.; Senewiratne, B.; Barnard, J. R.; Ohira, Y. <u>Am. J. Clin. Nutr.</u> 1977, 30, 910–17.
16. Edgerton, V. R.; Gardner, G. W.; Ohira, Y.; Gunawardena, K. A.; Senewiratne, <u>B. Brit. Med. J.</u> 1979, 2, 1546–49.
17. Ekblom, B.; Goldberg, A.; Gullbring, B. <u>J. Appl. Physiol.</u> 1972, 33, 175–80.
18. Woodson, R. D.; Wills, R. E.; Leufant, C. <u>J. Appl. Physiol.</u> 1978, 44, 36–43.
19. Buick, F. J.; Gledhill, A. B.; Foresi, A. B.; Sprint, L.; Meyers, E. C. <u>J. Appl. Physiol.</u> 1980, 48, 636–42.
20. Williams, M. H.; Wesseldine, S.; Somma, T.; Schuster, R. <u>Med. Sci. Sport Exercise</u> 1981, 13, 169–75.
21. Murray, J. F.; Gold, P.; Johnson, L. <u>Am. J. Physiol.</u> 1962, 203, 702–724.
22. Dallman, P. R.; Schwartz, H. C. <u>Pediatrics,</u> 1965, 35, 677–86.
23. Cusack. R. P.; Brown, W. D. <u>J. Nutr.</u> 1965, 86, 383–93.
24. Finch, C. A.; Miller, L. R.; Inandey, A. R.; Person, R.; Seiler, K.; Mackler, B. <u>J. Clin. Invest.</u> 1979, 58, 447–53.
25. Finch, C. A.; Gollnick, P. D.; Alastala, M. P.; Miller, L. R.; Dillman, E.; Mackler, B. <u>J. Clin. Invest.</u> 1979, 64, 129–37.
26. Hochacka, P.; French, C.; Guppy, M. In "Third International Symposium on Biochemistry of Exercise"; Landry, F., Orbay, W., eds.; Symposia Specialist: New York, 1978; p. 29.
27. Hollozsy, J. O.; Oscai, C. B. <u>Arch. Biochem. Biophys.</u> 1969, 130, 653–56.
28. McLane, J. A.; Fell, F. D.; McKay, R. H.; Winder, W. W.; Brown, E. B.; Holloszy, J. O. <u>Am. J. Physiol.</u> 1981, 241, C47–54.
29. Davies, K. J.; Maguire, J. J.; Dallman, P. R.; Brooks, G. A.; Packer, L. A. In "The Biochemistry and Physiology of Iron", Saltman, P.; Hegenauer, J., Eds., Elsevier Press: New York, 1982; p. 591
30. McDonald, R.; Hegenauer, J.; Sucec, A.; Saltman, P. <u>Eur. J. Appl. Physiol.</u> 1984, 52, 414–19.
31. Ohira, Y.; Hegenauer, J.; Saltman, P.; Edgerton, V. R. <u>Bio. Trace. Elem. Res.</u> 1982, 4, 45–56.
32. Nordin, B. E. C. In "Calcium, Phosphate, and Magnesium Metabolism"; Nordin, B. E. C. ed., Churchill Livingstone: London, 1976; p. 1.
33. Glimcher, M. J. In "Handbook of Physiology: Endocrinology"; Greep, R. O.; Astwood, E. B., Eds.; Vol. VII, American Physiological Society: Washington, D. C., 1976; p. 25.
34. Urist, M. R. In "The Biochemistry and Physiology of Bone 2nd Ed.", Bourne, G. H., Ed.; Academic Press: New York, 1976; p. 2.

35. Heaney, R. P. In "The Biochemistry and Physiology of Bone 2nd Ed."; Bourne, G. H., Ed.; Academic Press: New York, 1976; p. 106.
36. Vaughan, J. "The Physiology of Bone"; Claredon, Oxford, 1981.
37. Hoyle, G. Scientific American 1970, 222, 84-93.
38. Cohen, C. Scientific American 1975, 223, 36-45.
39. Robertson, W. G. In "Calcium, Phosphate and Magnesium Metabolism"; Nordin, B. E. C., Ed.; Churchill Livingstone: London, 1976; p. 113.
40. Curtis, B. A. J. Physiol. (London) 1963, 166, 75-86.
41. Luttgau, H. J. Physiol. (London) 1963, 168, 679-97.
42. Winegrad, S.; Shane, A. M. J. Gen. Physiol. 1962, 45, 371-94.
43. Heibrunn, L. V.; Wiercinski, F. J. J. Cell Comp. Physiol. 1947, 29, 15-32.
44. Huxley, A. F.; Niedergerke, R. Nature 1954, 173, 971-73.
45. Huxley, H. E.; Hanson, J. Nature 1954, 173, 973-76.
46. Hoyle, G.; Smyth, J. Comp. Biochem. Physiol. 1963, 10, 291-314.
47. Brostrom, C. O.; Hunkeler, F. L.; Krebs, E. G. J. Biol. Chem. 1971, 246, 1961-67.
48. Frankenhaeuser, B.; Hodgkin, A. L. J. Physiol. (London) 1957, 137, 218-44.
49. McLenna, H. "Synaptic Transmission"; Sanders: Philadelphia, 1970.
50. Malm, O. J. Scan. J. Clin. Lab. Invest. Suppl. 1958, 10, 1-289.
51. Wasserman, R. H.; Comar, C. L.; Nold, M. M. J. Nutr. 1956, 59, 371-83.
52. Helbock, H. J.; Forte, J. G.; Saltman, P. Biochem. Biophys. Acta 1966, 126, 81-93.
53. Condon, J. R.; Nassim, J. R.; Millard, F. J. C.; Hibe, A.; Stainthorpe, E. M. Lancet 1970, i, 1027-29.
54. Agnew, J. E.; Holdsworth, C. D. Gut 1971, 12, 973-77.
55. Albanese, A. A.; Edelson, A. H.; Woodhull, M. W.; Lorenzo, E. J.; Wein, E. H.; Orto, L. A. Nutr. Reports Inter. 1973, 8, 119-130.
56. Smith, E. L.; Reddan, W.; Smith, P. E. Med. Sci. Sport Exercise 1981, 13, 60-4.
57. Garn, S. M.; Rohmann, C. G.; Wagner, B. Fed. Proc. 1967, 26, 1729-36.
58. Smith, E. L. In "Internation Conference on Bone Mineral Measurement"; U. S. Department of HEW, Washington, D. C., 1973.
59. Heaney, R. P. Am. J. Med. 1962, 33, 188-200.
60. Riggs, B.; Ryan, R.; Wahner, N-S.; Mattox, V. J. Clin. Endo. Metab. 1973, 36, 1097-99.
61. Nilsson, B. E.; Westlin, N. E. Clin. Ortho. Rel. Res. 1971, 179-82.
62. Albright, F.; Smith, P. H.; Richardson, A. M. J. A. M. A., 1941, 114, 2465-74.
63. Mack, P. B.; LaChance, P. A.; Vose, G. P.; Vogt, F. B. Am. J. Roent. 1967, 100, 503-11.
64. Brewer, V.; Meyer, B. M.; Keele, S. J.; Hagan, R. D. Med. Sci. Sport Exercise 1983, 15, 445-49.
65. Saville, P. D.; Smith, R. E. Amer. J. Phys. Anthro. 1966, 25, 35-40.
66. Saville, P. D.; Whyte, M. P. Clin. Orthop. 1969, 65, 81-88.

67. Chavapil, M.; Bartos, D.; Bartos, F. <u>Gerontologia</u> 1973, 19, 263-77.
68. Kiishinen, A.; Heikkinen, <u>J. Appl. Physiol.</u> 1978, 44, 50-4.
69. Cuthberton, D. P. <u>Biochem. J.</u> 1929, 23, 1328-45.
70. Issekutz, B.; Blizzard, J. J.; Birkhead, N. C.; Rodahl, K. <u>J. Appl. Physiol.</u> 1966, 21, 1013-20.
71. Nordin, B. E. C.; Hodgkinson, A.; Peacock, M. <u>Clin. Orthop.</u> 1967, 52, 293-322.
72. Howard, J. E.; Parson, W.; Binghan, R. S. <u>Bull. Johns Hopkins Hosp.</u> 1945, 291-313.
73. Whedon, G. D.; Shorr, E. <u>J. Clin. Invest.</u> 1957, 36, 966-81.
74. McDonald, R. Unpublished data, 1984.
75. Bogert, L. J.; Kirkpatrick, E. E. <u>J. Biol. Chem.</u> 1922, 54, 375-86.
76. Shohl, A. T.; Sato, A. <u>J. Biol. Chem.</u> 1923, 58, 257-66.
77. Lemann, J.; Litzou, J. R.; Lennon, E. J. <u>J. Clin. Invest.</u> 1967, 46, 1318-28.
78. Greenberg, A. J.; McNamara, H.; McCrory, W. W. <u>J. Pedia.</u> 1966, 69, 610-18.
79. Walser, M. In "Renal Pharmacology"; Appleton-Century-Crofts: New York, 1971; p. 21.
80. Underwood, E. J. In "Trace Elements in Human and Animal Nutrition"; Academic Press: New York, 1977; p. 56.
81. O'Dell, B. L. In "Present Knowledge in Nutrition, 5th Ed."; Nutrition Foundation: Washington, D. C. 1984; p. 506.
82. Li, T-K.; Vallee, B. C. In "Modern Nutrition in Health and Disease, 6th Ed."; Goodhard, R. S.; Shils, M. E. Eds., Lea and Febiger: Philadelphia, 1980; p. 408.
83. Prasad, A. S. <u>Nutrition Reviews</u> 1983, 41, 197-208.
84. Underwood, E. J. In "Trace Elements in Human and Animal Nutrition"; Academic Press: New York, 1977; p. 196.
85. Sandstead, H. H.; Evans, G. W. In "Present Knowledge in Nutrition, 5th Ed."; Nutrition Foundation: Washington, D. C., 1984, p. 479.
86. Fell, B. F.; Mills, R. B.; Boyne, R. <u>Res. Vet. Sci.</u> 1965, 6, 10-14.
87. Gallagher, C. H.; Reeve, V. E. <u>Aust. J. Exp. Biol. Med. Sci.</u> 1971, 49, 21-31.
88. Davies, K. J.; Packer, L.; Brooks, G. A. <u>Arch. Biochem. Biophys.</u> 1982, 215, 260-265.
89. Strause, L.; Hegenauer, J.; Saltman, P.; Cone, R.; Resnick, D. Am. J. Clin. Nutr. Submitted, 1984.
90. Siegal, R. C.; Pinnell, S. R.; Markin, G. R. <u>Biochemistry</u> 1970, 9, 4486-90.
91. Gubler, C. J.; Cartwright, G. E.; Wintrobe, M. M. <u>J. Biol. Chem.</u> 1957, 224, 533-46.
92. Schloen, L. H.; Fernades, G.; Garofalo, J. A.; Good, R. A. <u>Clinical Bulletin</u> 1979, 9, 63-75.
93. Good, R. A.; Fernades, G.; Garofalo, J. A.; Cunningham-Rundles, C.; Iwata, J.; West, A. In "Clinical Biochemical and Nutritional Aspects of Trace Elements"; Prasad, A. S. Eds.; Alan R. Liss, Inc.: New York, 1982, p. 189.
94. Chandra, R. K.; Dayton, B. <u>Nutrition Research</u> 1982, 2, 721-33.
95. Prasad, A. S. <u>Nutrition Reviews</u> 1983, 41, 197-208.

96. Brummerstedt, E.; Flagstad, T.; Basse, A.; Andersen, E. Acta Pathol. Microbiol. Scand. 1971, 79, 686-88.
97. McCaffrey, R.; Smoler, D. F.; Baltimore, D. L. Proc. Nat. Acad. Sci. 1973, 70, 521-25.
98. De Pasquale-Jardiew, R.; Fraker, P. J. J. Nutr. 1979, 109, 1847-55.

RECEIVED April 19, 1985

Water and Electrolytes

John E. Greenleaf and Michael H. Harrison

Laboratory for Human Environmental Physiology, Biomedical Research Division, NASA Ames Research Center, Moffett Field, CA 94035

Under optimal conditions humans have been able to survive about 10 minutes without oxygen, up to 18 days without water, but nearly 60 days without food. Despite the fact that oxidation of nutrients produces water, there is a longer lasting supply of foodstuffs within the body than water. Part of the fatigue mechanism occurring during physical exercise can be attributed to fluid loss (dehydration) from the body and possibly to fluid-electrolyte shifts within the body. There is no adaptation to successive periods of dehydration and the performance of the strongest and fittest people will deteriorate rapidly with dehydration. When compared with the daily variability of many physico-chemical parameters, the least variability is found in body temperature, and plasma sodium, chloride, calcium, and osmolality (1). There is a close association between thermoregulation and the sodium, calcium, and osmotic concentration of the extracellular fluid; increases in plasma sodium concentration (hypernatremia) and plasma osmotic concentration (hyperosmotemia) tend to increase body temperature while hypercalcemia tends to decrease body temperature (2-4). The precise control of the concentration of these ions suggests that their functions are of major importance for optimal physiological homeostasis and survival of the organism.

In this paper we will discuss the anatomy of the fluid spaces in the body, the fluid shifts and losses during exercise and their effects on performance, and thirst and drinking during exercise with comments on carbohydrate ingestion.

Anatomy of Body Fluid Compartments

Total body water is arbitrarily divided into that contained within cells (cellular) and that located outside the cells (extracellular). The extracellular water is further divided into that contained within the vascular system excluding the erythrocytes (plasma), and that located outside the vascular system and outside the cells (interstitial fluid) (Figure 1).

Approximate volumes and percent of body weight of the various fluid compartments, and a daily water balance of a resting 80-kg man (5), are given in Tables I and II. With exercise, the sweat loss and beverage (fluid) intake would be greater. Oxidation of 1 gram of various foodstuffs would yield the following approximate water production (5): monosaccharides (glucose) = 0.6 g, disaccharides (sucrose) = 0.6 g, starch = 0.6 g, fat (lard) = 1.1 g, and protein = 0.4 g. The preformed volume of water would vary with the quantity and type of foodstuff metabolized (5). Its sources are the polymerization of glucose, condensation of amino acids, esterification of fats (glycerol), hydration of protein, and bound water (water of association); the latter source is 1 g of protein associated with 3 g H_2O, 1 g neutral fat with 0.1 g H_2O, and 1 g glycogen with 2.7 g H_2O.

Table I. Fluid Compartment Volumes of a Resting 80 kg Man*

Compartment	Volume, liters	Body weight, %
Extracellular:		
Plasma	4	5
Interstitial	19	24
Cellular	30	37
Total	53	66

*Modified from (5).

Table II. Daily Water Balance of a Resting 80 kg Man*

	Weight, grams	Percent
Input		
Beverage	1200	48
Food water (liquid)	1000	40
Oxidation water (metabolic)	250	10
Preformed water (metabolic)	50	2
Total	2500	100
Output		
Urine water	1400	56
Insensible water (vapor)	900	36
Fecal water	200	8
Sweat	0	0
Total	2500	100
Water balance (input-output)	0	

*Modified from (5).

Depending upon the quantity of fat in the body, body water in normal healthy people comprises 50% to 70% of the body weight. The higher the percentage of lean body mass, the higher the percentage of

water because lean mass (muscle) contains more water than fat tissue
(Table III). In the general population, the body water content aver-
ages about 61% (6). The half-life of body water molecules is about
12 days (7); the total water volume is regulated daily to within
±0.22% (±150 g) of the body weight (8), and plasma volume to within
±0.7% (±25 g) (9).

Table III. Weight and Water Content of Body Tissue From a
70.6 kg Man*

Tissue	Percent of body weight	Percent water content
Striated muscle	31.6	79.5
Skeleton	14.8	31.8
Adipose tissue	13.6	50.1
Skin	7.8	64.7
Lungs	4.2	83.7
Liver	3.4	71.5
Brain and spinal cord	2.5	73.3
Alimentary tract	2.1	79.1
Alimentary tract contents	0.8	---
Heart	0.7	73.7
Kidneys	0.5	79.5
Spleen	0.2	78.7
Pancreas	0.2	73.1
Bile	0.2	---
Teeth	0.1	5.0
Hair	0.1	---
Remaining tissues		
Liquid	3.7	93.3
Solid	13.5	70.4
Total Body	100.0	67.2

*Modified from (6).

Except for respiratory and dermal insensible water-vapor losses,
all remaining water lost by the body contains electrolytes, mainly
sodium and chloride. The normal cation and anion constituent composition of the fluid spaces is given in Table IV. In the extracellular fluid space, sodium is the major cation and chloride the major
anion. Those two ions constitute 95% of the extracellular fluid
osmolality. Changes in plasma sodium concentration reflect changes
in extracellular fluid volume. Potassium is the major cellular
cation and phosphates and proteins comprise the major anions. The
total cellular osmolality (175 + 135 = 310 mosmol/kg H_2O) is equal to
the total extracellular osmolality (155 + 155 = 310 mosmol/kg H_2O);
therefore, equal total osmotic concentrations are maintained between
two fluid compartments of widely different ionic contents (Table IV).

Exercise and Body Water

Exercise has two specific effects on body water. First, it alters
the distribution of water, colloids (protein), and crystalloids

Table IV. Normal Composition of Fluid Spaces in Man

Fluid space	Cations				Anions			
	Na$^+$	K$^+$	Other$^+$ Ca^{+2} + Mg^{+2}	Osmols$^+$	Cl$^-$	HCO^{-3}	Other$^-$ PO$_4^{-3}$ + PRO$^-$	Osmols$^-$
	mEq/l	mEq/l	mEq/l	mosmol/kg	mEq/l	mEq/l	mEq/l	mosmol/kg
Extracellular	142	5	8	155	103	27	25	155
Cellular	10	145	20	175	2	8	190	135
Total	152	150	28	330	105	35	215	290

(ions) within the body fluid compartments, Secondly, if sweat is
lost that is not replaced by fluid intake, the result is a decrease
in total body water content which, in hot environments, may be of
sufficient magnitude to reduce markedly the capacity for prolonged
exercise (10,11, Figure 2).

Fluid Shifts with Exercise. During exercise some plasma water is
lost (shifted) from the vascular compartment to the interstitial
compartment and to the cellular compartment of the active muscle
(12,13); at the same time fluid is shifted at a lower rate from the
interstitial compartment of inactive muscle to the vascular space
(14). The result is an absolute loss of plasma water (and electrolytes) that is directly proportional to the intensity of the exercise
(Figure 2). These transcompartmental fluid shifts occur as a result
of alterations in the balance of osmotic and hydrostatic forces
acting along and across the capillary networks of all tissues whose
blood flow is altered by exercise; e.g., muscle, skin, kidney, gut,
and liver. For exercise (cycling) performed in a seated position,
the fluid balance favors net capillary filtration which results in a
reduction of plasma volume or hemoconcentration (15). For exercise
performed in an upright position such as running, the hemoconcentration is often minimal (16) because the act of standing causes a substantial hemoconcentration; edema-preventing mechanisms, such as
increased interstitial fluid pressure, act to reduce the potential
for further hemoconcentration (17,18).
     Exercise at an intensity above 50% of peak working capacity is
usually accompanied by increased concentrations of plasma electrolytes; sodium, chloride, and especially potassium, with an accompanying increase in osmolality. There is, however, little change in
plasma electrolyte and osmotic concentrations at exercise levels
below 50% of the peak working capacity because the plasma filtrate is
isotonic with respect to existing plasma tonicity (19-21). At exercise levels above 50% of peak capacity, there is an exponential
increase in plasma sodium and osmolality that is associated with the
linear decrease in plasma volume (Figure 3) (20). Apart from an
increase in plasma-potassium concentration induced by the moderate
muscular contraction, which may be augmented by the breakdown of
glycogen to glucose (glycogenolytic activity) in active muscle, the

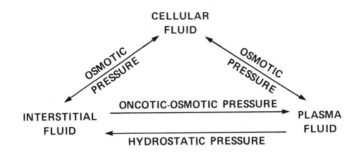

Figure 1. Cellular and extracellular (plasma and interstitial) fluid compartments.

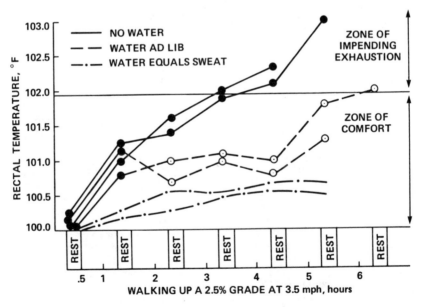

Figure 2. Effect of drinking water on rectal temperature levels during treadmill exercise (37.7°C dry-bulb temperature and 35-45% relative humidity) in one subject. From ref. 49 with permission.

elevations in plasma electrolyte and osmotic concentrations appear to
be a result of the transcompartmental fluid shifts. If moderate
dehydration is added to the stress of moderate exercise, especially
when performed in a hot environment, the elevation in plasma sodium
and osmotic concentrations can be sufficient to impair temperature
regulation (2,4).

Fluid shifts during exercise occur mainly as a result of
increased capillary filtration from the vascular compartment to the
interstitial space caused by the increases in hydrostatic and systemic blood pressures (13,21,22), with assistance from the increased
tissue osmolality (14,23) resulting from elevated muscle metabolism. The latter would tend to draw interstitial fluid into the
muscle cells (13) and, in conjunction with the shift of water from
inactive muscle, would increase tissue total pressure (Figure 1).
The reverse flux of fluid from the interstitial to the vascular space
(14) is caused by increased interstitial fluid pressure (12) and
increased plasma protein concentration (oncotic pressure),
hyperosmotemia, or both depending upon the intensity (above or below
50%-peak capacity) and duration of the exercise. Increased interstitial hydrostatic pressure and increased plasma osmotic pressures
retard the fluid shift from plasma to the interstitium. Equilibrium
is reached when interstitial pressure balances capillary filtration
pressure (24). After cessation of exercise, restitution of plasma
volume takes 40-60 minutes (21,22) unless significant dehydration is
present. The immediate post-exercise hyperosmotemia, the relative
hyperproteinemia, and the reduction in systemic blood pressure contribute to the restoration of plasma volume. The reduction in blood
pressure, which produces a fall in local hydrostatic pressure within
the capillaries of the previously active muscle, is probably the
single most important factor.

Consequences of Sweating. Sweating occurs during moderate exercise
levels in the cold as well as at higher environmental temperatures.
At low ambient temperatures a greater portion of the metabolic heat
production (depending upon exercise intensity and clothing) is dissipated by convection and radiation and a minor portion by evaporation
of sweat and respiratory water. As ambient temperature rises, the
portion of heat dissipated by convection and radiation decreases
progressively in concert with a proportional increase in the rate of
sweating and evaporative heat loss. The coordination of the rate of
heat loss between conduction, radiation, and evaporation is so precise that, for ambient dry-bulb temperatures between 5°C and 29°C,
the equilibrium level of core (rectal) temperature is related
directly to the intensity of the exercise load and is independent of
environmental temperature (25).

In cool environments the increase in metabolic heat production
and core temperature during exercise can be considered as an internal
thermal stress. The fluid shifts that occur during exercise in warm
and hot environments are modified by what can be considered as an
additional external thermal stress. Even under ideal (cool) climatic
conditions exercise is antihomeostatic, having the capability of
imposing simultaneous stresses upon nearly all the body's regulatory
systems. Prolonged exercise performed in hot conditions imposes a
particularly severe strain on the cardiovascular system which must
provide not only for the metabolic requirements of the working

muscles, but also for the dissipation of metabolic and environmental heat via regulation of the cutaneous circulation. Under the circumstance of great internal and external thermal stress, the dominant thermoregulatory mechanism is the production and evaporation of sweat.

For each milliliter of sweat evaporated, 2.4 kilojoules (0.58 kcal) of heat are lost from the body. During marathon runs in the heat, sweat rates may approach 2 liters per hour (26); if the body water lost is not replaced, dehydration occurs. Even in cool environments, where convection and radiation are the main avenues of heat dissipation, sweating may still result in significant dehydration because of the increase in core temperature. Therefore, appropriate fluid intake is an important requirement during prolonged exercise performed in cool environments as well as in the heat. Quantifying "prolonged" and "heat" is difficult, since the two are interactive. The heat produced by metabolism during intense exercise can exceed the absorption of extreme environmental heat by a factor of seven (27), but this level of metabolism can be sustained for only short periods of time. Rates of metabolic heat production exceeding 600 Watts, which is three times a severe environmental heat load, can be sustained for several hours by endurance athletes. A wet-bulb globe-temperature (WBGT) index [(0.7 × wet-bulb temp.) + (0.2 × black globe temp.) + (0.1 × dry-bulb temp.)] greater than 18°C (65°F) provides a condition for a potential risk of heat injury during exercise. Thus, the more intense and prolonged the exercise, the lower the safe WBGT index.

Sweat is composed of water and many solid substances, mainly the electrolytes sodium, potassium, and chloride (28). While loss of water and the ensuing increase in total body dehydration may become a medical problem, contrary to popular belief, the accompanying loss of electrolytes does not constitute a problem under most exercise and environmental situations as long as food consumption is normal. Sweat is much more dilute (hypotonic) than plasma (sweat = 0.4% solute, plasma = 0.9% solute). This hypotonicity increases in subjects who have undergone exercise training in the heat (acclimatization) (29). Consequently, sweating during exercise results in increases in plasma electrolyte and osmotic concentrations since proportionally more water than salt (electrolyte) is being lost in the sweat. But intravascular electrolyte content is also being decreased by losses in sweat. Once sweating ceases, and any body water deficit incurred is replaced by drinking pure water, the resulting intravascular electrolyte concentration will be decreased from the presweating level unless additional electrolytes are consumed. The best time to replace electrolytes lost during exercise is after exercise ceases because ingestion of electrolytes during exercise will add to the existing exercise-induced hyperosmolality. Drinking cold or warm water during exercise is more effective in attenuating the rise in core temperature than drinking an equal volume before exercise or providing artificial sweat by sponging the body with water during exercise (30). In addition, hypernatremia and hyperosmolality tend to inhibit sweating and evaporative heat loss (as does wet skin) and accentuate the already elevated core temperature (2,4,31).

There are circumstances when some electrolyte replacement is necessary, for example during repeated bouts of strenuous exercise

performed daily for many consecutive days, or when physical work or
exercise is performed continuously over a 12- to 24-hour period and
adequate rest periods and meals are not available. Muscle cramping
is a common response to salt (NaCl) depletion which usually can be
prevented by increasing salt intake. Heat cramp and the syndrome of
salt and/or water depletion heat exhaustion are commonly the result
of inappropriate levels of heat acclimatization and physical fitness
(32). The enhanced ability to conserve body sodium in sweat and
urine are major adaptive responses to heat acclimatization, and
excessive electrolyte depletion is usually a problem only during the
first few days of work in the heat. Further, it should be noted that
significantly increased salt intake during the first few days of heat
stress can inhibit the secretion of aldosterone (29), a hormone that
aids salt conservation by facilitating reabsorption of sodium in the
sweat glands and kidney tubules.

Provided that the diet is adequate, there is no substantial
evidence to suggest that loss of trace elements in sweat affects
nutritional status or exercise performance adversely (28). A possible exception is iron; the low level of bone marrow iron content
observed in some endurance-trained athletes (33) may be due to
excessive losses of as much as 40 micrograms of iron per 100 milliliters of sweat (34). Iron metabolism is discussed in more detail in
the chapter by McDonald and Saltman.

Dehydration and Exercise. Water loss corresponding to as little as
1% of the body weight leads to accentuated increases in body temperature and heart rate during exercise (Figure 4) (35). If water loss
approaches 4 to 5% of the body weight, the capacity for prolonged
work may be reduced by 20 to 30% (36). The adverse cardiovascular
and thermoregulatory effects of dehydration are partly a result of
reduction in plasma volume (hypovolemia) and an increase in plasma
osmolality. Hypovolemia also reduces stroke volume and cardiac output, and reduces the rate of heat loss by raising temperature thresholds for cutaneous vasodilatation and sweating (18). Thermal dehydration also elevates blood electrolytes and osmolality, and this too
reduces the sensitivity of heat-dissipation mechanisms independently
of any dehydration-induced reduction in plasma volume (3). Therefore, any factor which reduces plasma osmolality can only be advan-
tageous to the endurance athlete or worker performing in the heat--
another strong argument for not adding electrolytes to liquids consumed during exercise.

Dehydration also affects the plasma volume response to exercise. For example, during cycling in the heat, the magnitude of the
exercise hemoconcentration is greater when the cyclist is dehydrated
than when dehydration is prevented by drinking water (3). During
walking, the prevention of dehydration by water consumption increases
the tendency for hemodilution rather than for hemoconcentration
(37). Thus, preventing or minimizing dehydration improves performance during exercise through specific beneficial effects on both the
cardiovascular and thermoregulatory systems.

Heat Acclimatization and Endurance Training. Primary adaptive
responses to repeated intermittent exposure to exercise in the heat
are (1) chronic expansion of the plasma volume, (2) increased retention of body sodium, (3) increased capacity for sweating and, hence,

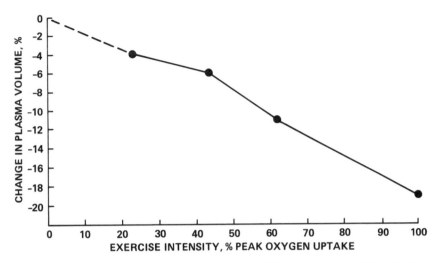

Figure 3. Plasma volume loss (shift) with increasing intensity of exercise. From ref. 71 with permission.

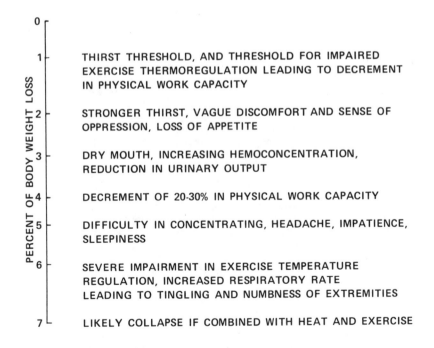

THIRST THRESHOLD, AND THRESHOLD FOR IMPAIRED EXERCISE THERMOREGULATION LEADING TO DECREMENT IN PHYSICAL WORK CAPACITY

STRONGER THIRST, VAGUE DISCOMFORT AND SENSE OF OPPRESSION, LOSS OF APPETITE

DRY MOUTH, INCREASING HEMOCONCENTRATION, REDUCTION IN URINARY OUTPUT

DECREMENT OF 20-30% IN PHYSICAL WORK CAPACITY

DIFFICULTY IN CONCENTRATING, HEADACHE, IMPATIENCE, SLEEPINESS

SEVERE IMPAIRMENT IN EXERCISE TEMPERATURE REGULATION, INCREASED RESPIRATORY RATE LEADING TO TINGLING AND NUMBNESS OF EXTREMITIES

LIKELY COLLAPSE IF COMBINED WITH HEAT AND EXERCISE

Figure 4. Adverse effects of dehydration.

for evaporative heat loss, and (4) some residual increase in
cutaneous blood flow (38,39). These responses provide for increased
heat dissipation during exercise, which allows core temperature to be
regulated at a lower level, and for reduced stress on the cardiovascular system after acclimatization. The practical importance of
expansion of the plasma volume which occurs with heat acclimatization
and endurance training remains controversial. Certainly it increases
the capacity of the cardiovascular system to maintain an adequate
blood flow to muscle and skin during exercise in the heat without
compromising either thermoregulation or regulation of blood pressure. On the other hand, the magnitude of the hemoconcentration
(hypovolemia) induced during cycling is greater after heat acclimatization. Corresponding data for running exercise are not available. Even though there is no adaptation to successive bouts of
dehydration, heat acclimatization seems to attenuate the adverse
effects of dehydration on the cardiovascular responses to heat and
exercise (40). Nothing can be gained, and much can be lost, by
performing prolonged exercise in a dehydrated condition, even for
acclimatized individuals. It should be emphasized that the physically conditioned endurance athlete needs as much and probably more
water than untrained people because of the increased sweating of the
athlete.

    Endurance exercise training, when carried out in cool environ-
ments, induces adaptive responses which are qualitatively similar to
those induced during heat acclimatization; i.e., increased sweat
rate, reduced heart rate, and increased plasma volume (41,42). When
heat acclimatization is induced by raising core temperature with
subjects at rest in a hot environment, these same adaptive responses
are enhanced to some degree (41,43). It has been observed that physically fit subjects do not exhibit these characteristic responses
when exposed to a standard acclimatization regimen involving intermittent walking exercise in a hot environment (44), suggesting that
they had already adapted in the same manner as acclimatized subjects. There appears to be some additive effect on the magnitude of
the adaptive responses between those induced by resting in the heat,
and exercising in cool and hot environments (45). The largest adaptive responses occur during the performance of moderate to heavy
exercise in the heat (18,41,42,46-48).

Thirst and Drinking During Exercise

Although it has been known for many years that dehydration and hypohydration impair physical performance, many people who engage in
exercise and exercise training may not know how serious that impairment can be or what to do about it, especially during competition
when they are confronted by rules that may prohibit or restrict
liquid consumption. A bewildering array of hydration drinks are
available commercially that bombard the individual with a variety of
claims, some of which border on the ludicrous. The truth is simple;
during exercise pure water is best. Although prevention of dehydration by replacement of all fluid losses would be the ideal procedure
for maximizing exercise performance in cool or hot environments (49),
in practice unfortunately, this full replacement is virtually impossible to achieve.

Stimuli for Drinking. Thirst stimulation and the act of drinking are basic physiological responses. The three major circumstances known to stimulate thirst and drinking are (1) a deficit of body water (hypohydration and hypovolemia), (2) an increase in the osmolality of the extracellular fluid volume (hyperosmolality and hyperosmotemia), and (3) consumption of dry food (prandial thirst) (50). These three factors can function independently, but they are often interactive; e.g., a hypovolemic subject is often hyperosmotic. In addition, the hormone angiotensin II acts as a stimulant for drinking (dipsogen) in animals, and possibly in man (51).

In humans experiencing thermally stressful conditions, the rate of voluntary fluid intake under optimal conditions for drinking, i.e., where cool palatable water or fruit juice (52) are readily accessible is, unfortunately, only about half the rate of water loss (51). Unless there is forced drinking, these stressed people are almost always in negative water balance. This condition is referred to as involuntary dehydration (53). The maximal strain on the fluid-electrolyte system occurs when a dehydrated person exercises in a hot environment. When the factors hydration-dehydration, exercise-rest, and hot-cool environments are separated, it is found that dehydration, exercise, and the hot environment all have greater inhibitory effects on drinking than their hydration, rest, and cool environment control conditions. Of these three stresses, heat exposure has the least inhibitory effect, prior dehydration has an intermediate effect, and moderate exercise per se has the greatest inhibitory effect on voluntary rehydration after stress-induced fluid loss (54). In spite of the differing nature of these various stimuli used to reduce body water, the rate of rehydration is the same when food and fluids are available ad libitum during a comfortable recovery period. The more stressful the total condition, the greater is the level of dehydration and the longer it takes to restore the lost water (54). In previously dehydrated men, forced fluid replacement over a 3-hour period of the fluid deficit failed to restore plasma volume and plasma osmolality to predehydration levels (55). The threshold for involuntary dehydration in hydrated subjects occurs with a water (sweat) loss of only 75 g/hr; with heat exposure the threshold is about 275 g/hr (54,56). This means that water losses below 75 g/hr and 275 g/hr are fully replaced by drinking voluntarily; above these thresholds they are not replaced fully. This is why drinking should be initiated before or immediately upon exposure to a stressful fluid-depleting situation before feelings of thirst arise (30); otherwise, significant levels of dehydration will occur that cannot be restored easily by drinking. Results from a recent study (51) indicate that heat acclimatization acts to reduce the level of involuntary dehydration during exercise in the heat by a progressively shortened time to the first drink, a threefold increase in the number of drinks per exposure, and a significant increase in the mean volume per drink. The result is that voluntary drinking can be increased comfortably from 450 ml/hr to 1000-1200 ml/hr (51). Thus, there appears to be an adaptive physiological response that allows one to increase fluid intake.

Water, Electrolyte, and Carbohydrate Replacement During Exercise. To help minimize the requirement for water replacement during exercise, adequate hydration should be attained before exercise commences.

Some forced drinking may be appropriate, but it must be planned care-
fully because the start of a competitive race is no time to have a
full bladder! Another method of storing water is by making use of
the 2.7 g of water of association with each gram of glycogen.
Increasing glycogen stores by consuming additional carbohydrates a
few days before exercise has the double advantage of providing additional reserves of both energy and water (36,57,58).

Enough has been said on the subject of electrolyte intake to
strongly suggest that the rule is to avoid salt (sodium and potassium). But there will be occasions when strict adherence to this
rule is inappropriate. Sometimes diet alone may not provide adequate
electrolytes or trace elements, for example when athletes perform
where customary foods are unavailable and local foods are unpal-
atable. If electrolyte supplements are necessary, they should be
taken with meals in conjunction with fluids. Under no circumstance
should salt be taken immediately before or during exercise, especially in hot environments when sweating and involuntary dehydration
are greatest and the rate of rise of hyperosmotemia is maximal. If
electrolyte consumption is necessary, for example when the exercise
must be performed over many hours in the heat (as in ultramarathon
events), then a very dilute salt solution (less than 0.5 grams per
100 milliliters of H_2O) is much better than salt tablets, which can
cause gastric irritation. Calcium should not be used in rehydration
drinks because it inhibits the normal hypervolemic response to fluid
ingestion (59). The ideal time for electrolyte supplementation is
after exercise when a sufficient amount of water can be taken to
dilute the salt to isotonicity (0.9 grams of NaCl per 100 milliliters
of H_2O), i.e., the normal concentration of plasma. Normally these
electrolyte supplements will be unnecessary as a balanced diet will
provide sufficient electrolytes and trace elements to restore any
temporary deficit.

Gastric emptying time (the normal maximal rate being about
600-800 ml/hr (60)) imposes a physiological limitation upon the rate
of fluid uptake into the circulatory system. Acute gastric discomfort usually arises when an attempt is made to drink large volumes of
liquid too quickly during exercise. A modest volume taken at fre-
quent intervals (100-125 ml or 4 ounces per 10 min) is usually all
that is comfortably possible, but the beneficial effect can be considerable. Water is absorbed from the stomach at a rate of about
2.6% of the ingested volume per minute, but at 20% of the ingested
amount per minute from the small intestine. Therefore, it is certainly the retention of fluid within the stomach that produces the
discomfort. The stomach can be envisioned essentially as a pump that
passes material into the duodenum (61). The rate of gastric emptying
increases in proportion to the volume ingested (60-62), and the addition of even small amounts of carbohydrates (monosaccharides and
disaccharides) has been reported to retard gastric emptying
(60,63-65). The addition of potassium chloride to a test meal slows
gastric emptying similarly to that induced by glucose, but the KCl is
more nauseating than glucose (65). Optimal gastric emptying occurs
when saline, of a concentration that is nearly isosmotic with the
plasma, is introduced into the stomach (61); hypertonic solutions
empty more slowly (61,66).

With prolonged exercise it may be necessary to provide additional carbohydrate energy sources since glycogen appears to be the

preferred substrate for energy production (67). Compared with the consumption of a normal mixed diet, consumption of a carbohydrate-enriched diet prior to exercise can result in significantly better running performance (68). Depletion of muscle glycogen by exercise and subsequent replenishment with enhanced carbohydrate feeding has also been reported to increase subsequent physical performance (69). Ingestion of a glucose polymer supplement during exercise increases endurance time at a work rate of 45% of the maximal capacity (70). Thus, carbohydrate feeding appears to enhance exercise performance, but, as with water and electrolytes, moderation is important to minimize the retardation effect on gastric emptying.

Summary

Deterioration of physical exercise performance due to dehydration begins when body weight decreases by about 1%. Unacclimatized humans under thermal and exercise stress will voluntarily drink at a rate of about half of the rate of their fluid losses even at low rates of fluid loss (275 ml/hr); the maximal rate of fluid intake is about 600-800 ml/hr, the normal maximal rate of gastric emptying. During the exercise-heat acclimatization procedure, the voluntary fluid intake can be increased from 450 ml/hr to 1000-1200 ml/hr with no adverse effects. Electrolyte supplementation in drinking fluid is not recommended during exercise bouts lasting less than 3 to 5 hours because the increased concentration of sodium in the plasma accentuates the hyperthermia. Electrolyte and carbohydrate supplementation is recommended during longer work or exercise periods, especially in hot environments, and when regular meals are not available. Thus, there has been no significant evidence that would change the conclusion of Pitts et al. in 1944 (49): "...in the case of well acclimatized young men whose daily diet is adequate, the best performance of intermittent work in the heat is to be achieved by replacing water loss hour by hour and salt loss meal by meal."

Literature Cited

1. Sargent, F., II; Weinman, K. (1963) Physiological variability in young men. In: Physiological Measurements of Metabolic Functions in Man (Consolazio, C.F., Johnson, R.E., and Pecora, L.J., eds.), p. 453, McGraw-Hill, New York, NY.
2. Greenleaf, J.E. (1979) Hyperthermia and exercise. In: Int. Rev. Physiol., Environ. Physiol. III, Vol. 20 (Robertshaw, D., ed.), p. 157, University Park Press, Baltimore, MD.
3. Harrison, M.H., Edwards, R.J. & Fennessy, P.A. (1978) Intravascular volume and tonicity as factors in the regulation of body temperature. J. Appl. Physiol.: Respirat. Environ. Exercise Physiol. 44, 69-75.
4. Kozlowski, S., Greenleaf, J.E., Turlejska, E. & Nazar, K. (1980) Extracellular hyperosmolality and body temperature during physical exercise in dogs. Am. J. Physiol. 239 (Regulatory Integrative Comp. Physiol. 8), R180-R183.
5. Johnson, R.E. (1964) Human nutritional requirements for water in long space flights. In: Nutrition in Space and Related Waste Problems (Helvey, T.C., ed.), p. 159, National Aeronautics and Space Administration, Washington, DC.

6. Oser, B.L. (ed.) (1965) Hawk's Physiological Chemistry.
    McGraw-Hill, New York, NY.
7. Schloerb, P.R., Friis-Hansen, B.J., Edelman, I.S., Solomon, A.K.
    & Moore, F.D. (1950) The measurement of total body water in the
    human subject by deuterium oxide dilution: with a consideration
    of the dynamics of deuterium distribution. J. Clin. Invest. 29,
    1296-1310.
8. Wolf, A.F. (1958) Thirst. Physiology of the Urge to Drink and
    Problems of Water Lack. C.C. Thomas, Springfield, IL.
9. Greenleaf, J.E., Convertino, V.A. & Mangseth, G.R. (1979)
    Plasma volume during stress in man: osmolality and red cell
    volume. J. Appl. Physiol.: Respirat. Environ. Exercise
    Physiol. 47, 1031-1038.
10. Adolph, E.F. & Associates (1947) Physiology of Man in the
    Desert. Interscience Publishers, Inc., New York, NY.
11. Dill, D.B., Bock, A.V., Edwards, H.T. & Kennedy, P.H. (1936)
    Industrial fatigue. J. Indust. Hyg. Toxicol. 18, 417-431.
12. Mohsenin, V. & Gonzales, R.R. (1984) Tissue pressure and plasma
    oncotic pressure during exercise. J. Appl. Physiol.: Respirat.
    Environ. Exercise Physiol. 56, 102-108.
13. Sjogaard, G. & Saltin, B. (1982) Extra- and intracellular water
    spaces in muscles of man at rest and with dynamic exercise. Am.
    J. Physiol. 243 (Regulatory Integrative Comp. Physiol. 12),
    R271-R280.
14. Lundvall, J., Mellander, S., Westling, H. & White, T. (1972)
    Fluid transfer between blood and tissue during exercise. Acta
    Physiol. Scand. 85, 258-269.
15. Harrison, M.H., Edwards, R.J. & Leitch, D.R. (1975) Effect of
    exercise and thermal stress on plasma volume. J. Appl. Physiol.
    39, 925-931.
16. Edwards, R.J. & Harrison, M.H. (1984) Intravascular volume and
    protein responses to running exercise. Med. Sci. Sports Exerc.
    16, 247-255.
17. Hagan, R.D., Diaz, F.J. & Horvath, S.M. (1978) Plasma volume
    changes with movement to supine and standing positions. J.
    Appl. Physiol.: Respirat. Environ. Exercise Physiol. 45,
    414-418.
18. Harrison, M.H. (1985) Effects of thermal stress and exercise on
    blood volume in humans. Physiol. Rev. 65, 149-209.
19. Convertino, V.A., Keil, L.C., Bernauer, E.M. & Greenleaf, J. E.
    (1981) Plasma volume, osmolality, vasopressin, and renin
    activity during graded exercise in man. J. Appl. Physiol.:
    Respirat. Environ. Exercise Physiol. 50, 123-128.
20. Convertino, V.A., Keil, L.C. & Greenleaf, J.E. (1983) Plasma
    volume, renin, and vasopressin responses to graded exercise
    after training. J. Appl. Physiol.: Respirat. Environ. Exercise
    Physiol. 54, 508-514.
21. Greenleaf, J.E., Convertino, V.A., Stremel, R.W., Bernauer,
    E.M., Adams, W.C. Vignau, S.R. & Brock, P.J. (1977) Plasma
    [Na$^+$], [Ca^{2+}], and volume shifts and thermoregulation during
    exercise in man. J. Appl. Physiol: Respirat. Environ. Exercise
    Physiol. 43, 1026-1032.

22. Greenleaf, J.E., Van Beaumont, W., Brock, P.J., Morse, J.T., & Mangseth, G.R. (1979) Plasma volume and electrolyte shifts with heavy exercise in sitting and supine positions. Am. J. Physiol. 236 (Regulatory Integrative Comp. Physiol. 5), R206-R214.

23. Mellander, S., Johansson, B., Gray, S., Jonsson, O., Lundvall, J., & Ljung, B. (1967) The effects of hyperosmolarity on intact and isolated vascular smooth muscle: Possible role in exercise hyperemia. Angiologica 4, 310-322.

24. Smith, E.E., Guyton, A.C., Manning, R.D., & White, R.J. (1976) Integrated mechanisms of cardiovascular response and control during exercise in the normal human. Prog. Cardiovasc. Dis. 18, 421-443.

25. Nielsen, M. (1938) Die Regulation der Körpertemperatur bei Muskelarbeit. Scand. Arch. Physiol. 79, 193-230.

26. Maron, M.B. & Horvath, S.M. (1978) The marathon: a history and review of the literature. Med. Sci. Sports 10, 137-150.

27. Mitchell, J.W. (1977) Energy exchanges during exercise. In: Problems with Temperature Regulation during Exercise (Nadel, E.R., ed.), pp. 11-26, Academic Press Inc., NY.

28. Robinson, S. & Robinson, A.H. (1954) Chemical composition of sweat. Physiol. Rev. 34, 202-220.

29. Davies, J.A., Harrison, M.H., Cochrane, L.A., Edwards, R.J. & Gibson, T.M. (1981) Effect of saline loading during heat acclimatization on adrenocortical hormone levels. J. Appl. Physiol.: Respirat. Environ. Exercise Physiol. 50, 605-612.

30. Gisolfi, C.V. & Copping, J.R. (1974) Thermal effects of prolonged treadmill exercise in the heat. Med. Sci. Sports 6, 108-113.

31. Greenleaf, J.E. & Castle, B.L. (1971) Exercise temperature regulation in man during hypohydration and hyperhydration. J. Appl. Physiol. 30, 847-853.

32. Leithead, C.S. (1964) Disorders of water and electrolyte balance. In: Heat Stress and Heat Disorders (Leithead, C.S. & Lind, A.R., authors), pp. 141-177, F.A. Davis Company, Philadelphia, PA.

33. Ehn, L., Carlmark, B. & Höglund, S. (1980) Iron status in athletes involved in intense physical activity. Med. Sci. Sports Exerc. 12, 61-64.

34. Vellar, O.D. (1968) Studies on sweat losses of nutrients. I. Iron content of whole body sweat and its association with other sweat constituents, serum iron levels, hematological indices, body surface area, and sweat rate. Scand. J. Clin. Lab. Invest. 21, 157-167.

35. Ekblom, B., Greenleaf, C.J., Greenleaf, J.E. & Hermansen, L. (1970) Temperature regulation during exercise dehydration in man. Acta Physiol. Scand. 79, 475-483.

36. Olsson, K.-E. & Saltin, B. (1971) Diet and fluids in training and competition. Scand. J. Rehab. Med. 3, 31-38.

37. Sawka, M.N., Francesconi, R.P., Pimental, N.A. & Pandolf, K.B. (1984) Hydration and vascular fluid shifts during exercise in the heat. J. Appl. Physiol.: Respirat. Environ. Exercise Physiol. 56, 91-96.

38. Greenleaf, J.E. & Greenleaf, C.J. (1970) Human acclimation and acclimatization to heat: a compendium of research. NASA Tech. Memo. X-62,008, 1-188.

39. Sciaraffa, D., Fox, S.C., Stockmann, R. & Greenleaf, J.E.
     (1980) Human acclimation and acclimatization to heat: a
     compendium of research (1968-1978). NASA Tech. Memo. 81181,
     1-102.
40. Sawka, M.N., Toner, M.M., Francesconi, R.P. & Pandolf, K.B.
     (1983) Hypohydration and exercise: effects of heat
     acclimation, gender, and environment. J. Appl. Physiol.:
     Respirat. Environ. Exercise Physiol. 55, 1147-1153.
41. Convertino, V.A., Greenleaf, J.E. & Bernauer, E.M. (1980) Role
     of thermal and exercise factors in the mechanism of
     hypervolemia. J. Appl. Physiol.: Respirat. Environ. Exercise
     Physiol. 48, 657-664.
42. Shvartz, E., Bhattacharya, A., Sperinde, S.J., Brock, P.J.,
     Sciaraffa, D., Haines, R.F. & Greenleaf, J.E. (1979)
     Deconditioning-induced exercise responses as influenced by heat
     acclimation. Aviat. Space Environ. Med. 50, 893-897.
43. Fox, R.H., Goldsmith, R., Kidd, D.J. & Lewis, H.E. (1963)
     Acclimatization to heat in man by controlled elevation of body
     temperature. J. Physiol. (London) 166, 530-547.
44. Greenleaf, J.E. (1964) Lack of artificial acclimatization to
     heat in physically fit subjects. Nature 203, 1072.
45. Gisolfi, C. & Robinson, S. (1969) Relations between physical
     training, acclimatization, and heat tolerance. J. Appl.
     Physiol. 26, 530-534.
46. Convertino, V.A., Shvartz, E., Haines R.F., Bhattacharya, A.,
     Sperinde, S.J., Keil, L.C. & Greenleaf, J.E. (1977) Heat
     acclimation and water-immersion deconditioning: fluid and
     electrolyte shifts with tilting. Aerospace Med. Asso.
     Preprints, 13-14.
47. Senay, L.C., Mitchell, D. & Wyndham, C.H. (1976) Acclimatiza-
     tion in a hot humid environment: body fluid adjustments. J.
     Appl. Physiol. 40, 786-796.
48. Harrison, M.H., Edwards, R.J., Graveney, M.J., Cochrane, L.A., &
     Davies, J.A. (1981) Blood volume and plasma protein responses
     to heat acclimatization in humans. J. Appl. Physiol.:
     Respirat. Environ. Exercise Physiol. 50, 597-604.
49. Pitts, G.C., Johnson, R.E. & Consolazio, F.C. (1944) Work in
     the heat as affected by intake of water, salt and glucose. Am.
     J. Physiol. 142, 253-259.
50. Adolph, E.F. (1967) Regulation of water intake in relation to
     body water content. In: Handbook of Physiology, Section 6:
     Alimentary Canal, Vol. 1, Control of food and water intake
     (Code, C.F., ed.), p. 163, American Physiological Society,
     Washington, DC.
51. Greenleaf, J.E., Brock, P.J., Keil, L.C. & Morse, J.T. (1983)
     Drinking and water balance during exercise and heat acclima-
     tion. J. Appl. Physiol.: Respirat. Environ. Exercise Physiol.
     54, 414-419.
52. Sohar, E., Gilat, A.T., Tennenbaum, J. & Nir, M. (1961)
     Reduction of voluntary dehydration during effort in hot envi-
     ronments. J. Med. Asso. Israel 60, 319-323.
53. Greenleaf, J.E. (1966) Involuntary hypohydration in man and
     animals: a review. NASA Special Publication 110, 1-34.
54. Greenleaf, J.E. & Sargent, F., II (1965) Voluntary dehydration
     in man. J. Appl. Physiol. 20, 719-724.

55. Costill, D.L. & Sparks, K.E. (1973) Rapid fluid replacement following thermal dehydration. J. Appl. Physiol. 34, 299-303.

56. Rothstein, A., Adolph, E.F. & Wills, J.H. (1947) Voluntary dehydration. In: Physiology of Man in the Desert (Adolph, E.F. & Associates, eds.), p. 254, Interscience, New York, NY.

57. Costill, D.L., Bennett, A., Branam, G. & Eddy, D. (1973) Glucose ingestion at rest and during prolonged exercise. J. Appl. Physiol. 34, 764-769.

58. Krzentowski, G., Jandrain, B., Pirnay, F., Mosora, F., Lacroix, M., Luyckx, A.S. & Lefebvre, P.J. (1984) Availability of glucose given orally during exercise. J. Appl. Physiol.: Respirat. Environ. Exercise Physiol. 56, 315-320.

59. Greenleaf, J.E. & Brock, P.J. (1980) Na^+ and Ca^{2+} ingestion: plasma volume-electrolyte distribution at rest and exercise. J. Appl. Physiol.: Respirat. Environ. Exercise Physiol. 48, 838-847.

60. Costill, D.L. & Saltin, B. (1974) Factors limiting gastric emptying during rest and exercise. J. Appl. Physiol. 37, 679-683.

61. Hunt, J.N. & Knox, M.T. (1968) Regulation of gastric emptying. In: Handbook of Physiology, Section 6: Alimentary Canal, Vol. IV, Motility (Code, C.F., ed.), p. 1917, American Physiological Society, Washington, DC.

62. Erskine, L. & Hunt, J.N. (1981) The gastric emptying of small volumes given in quick succession. J. Physiol. (London) 313, 335-341.

63. Elias, E., Gibson, G.J., Greenwood, L.F., Hunt, J.N. & Tripp, J.H. (1968) The slowing of gastric emptying by monosaccharides and disaccharides in test meals. J. Physiol. (London) 194, 317-326.

64. Coyle, E.F., Costill, D.L., Fink, W.J. & Hoopes, D.G. (1978) Gastric emptying rates for selected athletic drinks. Res. Quart. 49, 119-124.

65. Barker, G.R., Cochrane, G.M., Corbett, G.A., Hunt, J.N. & Roberts, S.K. (1974) Actions of glucose and potassium chloride on osmoreceptors slowing gastric emptying. J. Physiol. (London) 237, 183-186.

66. Lee, P.R., Code, C.F. & Scholer, J.F. (1955) The influence of varying concentrations of sodium chloride on the rate of absorption of water from the stomach and small bowel of human beings. Gastroenterology 29, 1008-1015.

67. Ahlborg, B., Bergström, J., Ekelund, L.-G. & Hultman, E. (1967) Muscle glycogen and muscle electrolytes during prolonged physical exercise. Acta Physiol. Scand. 70, 129-142.

68. Karlsson, J. & Saltin, B. (1971) Diet, muscle glycogen, and endurance performance. J. Appl. Physiol. 31, 203-206.

69. Saltin, B. & Hermansen, L. (1967) Glycogen stores and prolonged severe exercise. In: Nutrition and Physical Activity (Blix, G., ed.), p. 32, Almqvist & Wiksells, Uppsala, Sweden.

70. Ivy, J.L., Miller, W., Dover, V., Goodyear, L.G., Sherman, W.M.,
     Farrell, S. & Williams, H. (1983) Endurance improvement by
     ingestion of a glucose polymer supplement. Med. Sci. Sports
     Exerc. 15, 466-471.
71. Greenleaf, J.E. (1982) The body's need for fluids. In:
     Nutrition and Athletic Performance (Haskell, W., Scala, J. &
     Whittam, J., eds.), p. 34, Bull Publishing Co., Palo Alto, CA.

RECEIVED March 15, 1985

Aerobic Exercise and Body Composition

Donald K. Layman[1] and Richard A. Boileau[2]

[1]Department of Foods and Nutrition, Division of Nutritional Sciences, University of Illinois, Urbana, IL 61801
[2]Department of Physical Education, Division of Nutritional Sciences, University of Illinois, Urbana, IL 61801

Body composition is a term used to characterize the relative constituents of the body. In the most general sense, the concept of body composition partitions the organism into fat and fat-free body components. These components are of particular importance because of their relationship to obesity which is one of the most compelling problems in nutrition and health in western societies.

Obesity is the accumulation of excess fat and, thus, is characterized by overfatness as opposed to simply overweight. To demonstrate the magnitude of obesity as a health problem, it has been estimated that adult Americans carry 2.3 billion pounds of excess fat (1). While little agreement on a precise definition of obesity can be found, useful but arbitrary standards are fat contents in excess of 20-25% of body weight for males and 25-30% for females. Using these figures, the prevalence of obesity has been estimated as 25-50% of the adult American population (2,3). Further, the prevalence of childhood obesity has been estimated to range from 5 to 30% in developed countries (4,5). In fact, the identification of obesity in childhood has become an important aspect of the revised Health-Related Fitness Test (6) given nationally to school children. The recent 1985 National Children and Youth Fitness Study (7) shows a continuing pattern of increasing fatness based on skinfold thickness measures in school children relative to data collected throughout the 1960's as part of the National Health Examination Survey (8,9).

While the direct effect of being obese on increased morbidity and mortality is difficult to assess, obesity has been designated as a significant health problem based on its statistical association with the increased risks of developing heart disease, hypercholesterolemia, hypertriglyceridemia, cancer, arthritis, hypertension, diabetes mellitus, and gout (10). There is also an increased risk related to the administration of anesthetics during surgery (11) and obesity is known to contribute to pulmonary stress (12).

It is generally accepted that the primary etiology of obesity concerns problems of energy balance as a consequence of nutritional excess and physical inactivity with less than 1% of cases associated with endocrine dysfunction (13). Changes in body weight or body composition depend on the relationship of energy intake to energy

0097-6156/86/0294-0125$06.00/0
© 1986 American Chemical Society

expenditure. This relationship, which is usually referred to as
energy balance, is positive when intake exceeds expenditure.
Positive energy balance produces increases in body weight, body fat,
or both. Weight loss occurs when expenditure exceeds intake. While
the energy balance relationship is clear, application of the concept
has not proven to be straightforward or easy.

The components of energy balance are intake, which is the
consumption of food, and expenditure, which is a combination of
basal metabolism (the energy expended at rest), specific dynamic
action (the energy expended in digestion, absorption, and
assimilation of nutrients after a meal), and exercise. Of the
components of this equation only intake and exercise can be
voluntarily altered. Thus for an individual to alter body weight or
composition requires changes in intake and/or exercise. Most
attempts to alter body weight involve caloric restriction or
dieting. While it is clear that caloric restriction will cause
weight loss, the data show that the majority of individuals losing
weight will regain some or all of the lost weight (14). Further, as
will be discussed later, little or no improvements may have occurred
in body composition. On the expenditure side of energy balance,
exercise is viewed by many as a critical factor in determining body
weight. While others believe that moderate, aerobic exercise
produces an insignificant expenditure of calories.

This chapter will review the relative contributions of exercise
and food intake to changes in body weight and more specifically body
composition. The emphasis of this chapter is on exercise as a
modality for fat reduction and fat-free weight maintenance with the
focus on aerobic exercise which has greater potential to modify body
composition due to larger effects on energy balance. The first
section reviews the effects of aerobic exercise on body composition
in humans. The second section addresses techniques for measurement
of body composition and limitations of these measurements in
humans. The third section examines the use of experimental animals
for studies of exercise and body composition, and the fourth section
examines the interactions of diet and exercise.

Effect of Aerobic Exercise on the Body Composition of Humans

Exercise represents the most variable factor on the expenditure side
of the energy balance equation. It is possible to increase the
energy expenditure 10-20 fold at peak exercise levels. Not only is
the metabolic rate increased during exercise, but the calorigenic
effect of exercise may remain significantly elevated for several
hours after exercise both in terms of recovery energy expenditure
(15) and appetite supression (16). On the other hand, the use of
exercise as treatment for body weight modification and fat loss has
been criticized on at least two counts. First, there is the belief
that caloric consumption associated with moderate aerobic exercise
is insignificant when compared to the much publicized semistarvation
diets. There is also the belief that exercise stimulates the
appetite so that any caloric deficit effected by exercise is offset
by increased food intake. Research to answer these and other
questions has not been convincing and certainly not definitive.
While one can generally conclude that exercise alone evokes a modest
modification in body composition, existing human research has been

plagued by the lack of controlled studies with respect to research design, quantification of energy intake and output, and methodological considerations in body composition assessment. In addition, most human research has been limited to relatively short-term studies due to problems associated with adherence, whereas the energetics of exercise would suggest that physiologically significant changes in body composition can only be accomplished through long-term programs. For example, a typical exercise program consisting of 30 minutes of exercise per session, 3 days per week may only increase caloric expenditure by 600-900 Kcal per week, a rate equivalent to a one pound fat loss every 4-5 weeks attributable solely to exercise.

The evidence suggesting that exercise is a significant factor in controlling and modifying human body composition has come from both comparative and experimental research designs. When physically active individuals, such as athletes or those involved in heavy physical labor, are compared to the more sedentary, the leanness to fatness ratio is invariably higher in active individuals. The normal range of relative fatness is 15-20% body weight for males and 20-25% for females. On the other hand, the range for athletic groups is normally 5-15% fat for males and 10-20% for females. Descriptions of the body composition characteristics of various male and female athletic groups have been provided in other reviews (17,18). It must be noted, however, that while cross-sectional comparisons of physically active to inactive groups suggest that exercise influences an increase in the leanness to fatness ratio, this interpretation must be tempered by consideration that lean individuals more frequently select or are selected to participate in physically demanding activities.

Interpretation of the experimental evidence concerning the effect of exercise on human body composition must also be viewed conservatively since only infrequently are control groups employed, ad libitum dietary practices are assumed to remain constant but are rarely monitored over the duration of the experiment and often a mismatch exists between exercise energy expenditure and body composition changes. The latter concern has been previously reported by Grande (19), Moody et al. (20), Wilmore et al. (21), and Boileau et al. (22). In these studies, the energy equivalent of fat reduction and FFB gain far exceeded the energy expended in exercise. This problem is likely multifaceted and may be related to inadvertent dietary caloric reduction, inaccurate estimation of exercise caloric expenditure, change in normal physical activity habits, or body composition methodological considerations.

In spite of the aforementioned problems in conducting body composition research on humans, there is convincing evidence to suggest that exercise is a significant factor in body weight control and fat reduction in nonobese and mildly obese individuals. However, when compared to animal data, the relative effects in humans appear at best to be modest. Further, there is general consensus that in severe obesity exercise alone is an insufficient treatment (23,24).

Several reviews have addressed the effect of aerobic exercise on body weight and composition modification (18,25,26,27). A summary of 32 studies involving adult males, adult females, and children is presented in Table I. The studies ranged from 8 to 20

Table I. Summary of the Effect of 8-20 Weeks of Aerobic
Exercise on Changes in Body Composition[1]

Group		Body Wt. (kg)	%Fat	Fat (kg)	FFB (kg)
Males	X	-1.2	-1.7	-1.7	0.4
(24 sample	SD	1.1	1.2	1.3	1.1
groups)					
Females	X	-1.9	-3.3	-2.9	1.0
(7 sample	SD	2.3	3.3	2.6	1.7
groups)					
Children	X	-1.6	-2.6	-2.1	0.5
(10 sample	SD	3.7	3.3	2.9	1.1
groups)					

[1]This table was constructed from a summary of data presented by
Wilmore (18) which included 25 studies of 8-20 weeks' duration. The
data for children include seven studies and were summarized from
Boileau et al. (27).

weeks' duration and, in general, training exceeded 30 minutes per
session with an average frequency of 3 days per week. The mode of
aerobic exercise consisted mostly of walking, jogging, running, and
bicycling. While relatively large variations can be seen among the
studies, a mean body weight reduction of 1.2, 1.9, and 1.6 kg was
observed for adult males, adult females, and children, respectively.
As expected in aerobic exercise, fat loss exceeded body weight loss
suggesting that the FFB was at least maintained. This is significant
since dietary restriction alone often leads to loss of body protein
and FFB (28). It is interesting that the 1.7 kg fat loss and 0.4 kg
FFB gain observed across the adult male studies represents an
expenditure of 15000 Kcal which is roughly equivalent to a moderate
aerobic exercise program of 10-15 weeks' duration.

While these studies lead to the conclusion that exercise evokes
a modest body weight and fat loss while maintaining the FFB, the
combination of moderate dietary caloric reduction and moderate
exercise energy expenditure may provide the optimal response. Zuti
and Golding (29) studied three body composition modification
programs including dietary caloric reduction (500 Kcal/day),
exercise (500 Kcal/day), and a combination of diet (250 Kcal/day)
and exercise (250 Kcal/day) in adult women judged to be 9-18 kg
overweight. The body weight decrease was similar among the groups
ranging from 4.5 to 5.5 kg during the program. Most of the weight
loss was accounted for by fat loss which was 4.2, 5.7, and 6.0 kg
for the diet, exercise, and combination groups, respectively. Fat
loss in the exercise and combination groups was similar but
significantly more than the diet group. Also, the exercise and
combination groups maintained their FFB gaining 0.5 and 0.9 kg,
respectively, whereas the diet group lost 1.1 kg of FFB. Clearly,
the maintenance of FFB appears to be an advantage provided by
exercise and needs to be considered an important aspect among the
various obesity treatment modalities.

Measurements of Body Composition

Measurements of body composition consist of direct and indirect
methods. Direct methods include measures of body protein, water,
fat, and ash (minerals). An alternative direct approach is
measurement of individual tissue weights. While these methods are
unambiguous and preferred, they are generally limited to studies
with animals. In non-sacrificial beings, direct determinations of
tissue weights are impossible, and determinations of body
composition are restricted to use of indirect, noninvasive methods.

Human body composition assessment relies on indirect
measurement techniques. Validation of these techniques is limited
to direct analysis of 4 or 5 adult cadavers, depending on the
measurement method (30,31). The measurement techniques most often
employed include densitometry, hydrometry, ^{40}K by gamma-ray
spectrometry, and anthropometry. The methodology of these
techniques has been reviewed for their use in children and adults in
several reports (17,26,32,33). Moreover, technological advances
have provided several additional techniques such as neutron
activation analysis (34) and other promising but as yet unvalidated
approaches, including total body impedance (35), electrical
conductivity (36), and nuclear magnetic resonance imagery (37).

A primary methodological consideration in the use of the
indirect techniques is the compositional model of the body. Several
models have been proposed including: a four-compartment system (28)
consisting of bone mineral, cells, and extracellular water as the
energy utilizing component plus fat as the energy storage component;
a three-component model (38) including fat, muscle, and a remainder
mass (muscle free lean); and two-component models consisting of
either fat-free body (32) or lean body mass (LBM) (39) and fat. The
conceptual difference between the fat-free body weight and lean body
mass models is that LBM includes essential fat. The two-component
model is used almost exclusively and data are derived from the
measurement methods mentioned above. Since densitometry is
considered the standard against which other techniques are compared
and validated, discussion here is limited to application of the two-
component model using the densitometric method for estimation of
body composition.

Body density (D_B) is the ratio of body weight (BW_{air}) to body
volume. Body volume can be measured by water displacement or helium
dilution, but the method of choice is underwater weighing (BW_{H2O})
with corrections for the density of water (DH_{H2O}) and residual lung
volume (RV) (40). Density is then estimated as follows:

$$D_B = \frac{BW_{air}}{\left[\dfrac{BW_{air} - BW_{H2O}}{D_{H2O}} \right] - RV}$$

When the two-component system is applied to the densitometric
estimation of fat and fat-free body, certain critical assumptions
must be made: (1) the densities of fat and FFB are known and
additive; (2) the densities of the FFB components (e.g., water,

mineral, and protein) are relatively constant within and among
individuals; (3) the proportion of each FFB component is relatively
constant within and among individuals with respect to the total FFB;
and (4) the individual being assessed differs only from a standard
"reference man" in the amount of depot fat possessed. Using these
assumptions, Morales et al. (41) described the following
mathematical model for the relationship of D_B to the fat and the
components of fat-free body:

$$\frac{1}{D_B} = \frac{f}{D_f} + \frac{w}{D_w} + \frac{m}{D_m} + \frac{p}{D_p}$$

where f, w, m, and p are the fractions of fat, water, mineral, and
protein, respectively, and D_f, D_w, D_m, and D_p the densities
of each component.

The relationship between body fat content (F_f) and body
density has been described by Siri (42) assuming the densities of
fat and FFB to be 0.900 gm/cc and 1.100 gm/cc, respectively:

$$F_f = \frac{4.95}{D_B} - 4.50$$

The assumption of FFB constancy both within an individual and among
individuals is, at best, only tenable within selected phases of the
life cycle and valid within sex and racial groups (43,44). Evidence
during growth and maturation suggests that the FFB is chemically
"immature" with the water content higher (45,46,47) and the mineral
content lower (48,49) than adult levels. Since water constitutes a
high percentage of the FFB but a relatively low density (0.9934
gm/cc at 37°C) and mineral a low percentage of the FFB but a high
density (3.0 gm/cc) with respect to overall FFB density, the
accepted value of 1.10 gm/cc generated for the adult model is likely
not applicable to the growing individual. This suggests that the
FFB density is lower and may range from 1.070 to 1.100 gm/cc during
growth and development (49,50).

There is also evidence that the FFB density may be altered in
the later stages of the aging continuum. Table II presents
estimates of change in the FFB density throughout the life cycle.
While these data are incomplete, the trend suggests that a primary
assumption in the use of densitometric analysis for assessment of
body composition may not be tenable. It is well known that there is
bone mineral loss with aging (52) which is particularly evident in
the postmenopausal female. This loss is at least one factor
affecting alterations in the relative proportions of the FFB
constituents. The extent to which water and protein change with
aging both in relative and absolute amounts is also an important
consideration. The magnitude of these changes and, thus, the change
in FFB density needs to be more definitively described in future
research so that accurate estimates of body fat and fat-free body
can be made.

Not only is the densitometric estimation of body composition
affected by life cycle changes in the composition of the FFB so,
too, are other methods which are based on similar assumptions. For

Table II. Estimated Changes in Density of the Fat-Free Body
Throughout the Life Cycle for Males[a]

Age	N	%FFB	Density FFB gm/cc
5	--	85.4	1.078
10	39	83.5	1.082
12	21	83.6	1.091
15	52	85.1	1.096
20-29	45	83.1	1.106
40-49	34	69.7	1.092
50-59	30	68.7	1.089
60-69	25	68.4	1.085
70-79	21	70.4	1.085

[a]Estimates of the fat-free body density were made from density and
body water data [Siri (42)]. The data were derived from Fomon et
al. (49) for the 5-year-old male, Boileau et al. (50) for the 10-
to 29-year-old males, and Norris et al. (51) for the 40- to
79-year-old males.

example, changes in the hydration of the FFB and potassium content
of the FFB require fundamental adjustments in the "assumed"
constants for estimation of body composition by hydrometry and ^{40}K
spectrometry.

Perhaps the most popular clinical method utilized to estimate
body fat employs the skinfold caliper to measure subcutaneous fat.
The method is based on the fact that a relatively large proportion
of total body fat lies just below the skin. Skinfold thickness is
inversely related to body density. Based on the relationship
between subcutaneous fat and body density, skinfold thickness
measures are used to estimate body density via regression
equations. While this relationship can provide accurate estimates
of body composition, the reliability depends on the accuracy of the
skinfold measurements, the quality of the regression equations, and
the validity of the density values. Because of these factors the
relationship of skinfold thickness to body density appears to change
throughout the life cycle (53); therefore, the regression equation
employed must be valid for the sample group being assessed.

Effect of Aerobic Exercise on the Body Composition of Experimental Animals

While it is critical to study the effects of aerobic exercise on
humans, the limitations of body composition methodology plus the
even more difficult problems of controlling and defining dietary
intake and total physical activity make use of animal models
essential. Use of experimental animals allows for control of diet
and exercise plus precise characterization of experimental groups
(i.e., age, sex, weight, and genetic background). Further,
experimental conditions including caloric intake, length of study,
and exercise intensity and duration can be modified over a larger
range. These factors make experiments with animals important for
the evaluation and understanding of data from studies with humans.

Under controlled conditions of dietary intake and daily
exercise, it is clear that aerobic exercise reduces body weight in
experimental animals (54,55,56). To illustrate this point, we have
presented data from our laboratory using a moderate aerobic exercise
program [approximately 75% VO_{2max} (57)] in Table III. Male rats

Table III. Body and Tissue Weights After 12 Weeks
of Exercise Training

Tissues	Units	Sedentary	Trained
Body weight	(g)	578 ± 10.3	493 ± 7.9 *
Organs			
Heart	(g)	1.23 ± 0.26	1.20 ± 0.04
Liver	(g)	11.6 ± 0.4	11.3 ± 0.1
Adrenals	(mg)	24 ± 1	27 ± 1 *
Skeletal Muscles			
Soleus	(mg)	163 ± 6	164 ± 5
Plantaris	(mg)	492 ± 24	449 ± 8
Gastrocnemius	(g)	2.35 ± 0.05	2.24 ± 0.04
Psoas	(g)	1.45 ± 0.04	1.42 ± 0.04
Adipose Tissues			
Perirenal	(g)	3.63 ± 0.16	1.86 ± 0.16*
Epididymal	(g)	2.88 ± 0.10	1.91 ± 0.09*
Inguinal	(g)	5.19 ± 0.24	3.18 ± 0.13*

Values are Means + SEM, n = 21, * $p < 0.05$.
(Quig and Layman, unpublished.)

8 weeks old and weighing 200 g were trained 5 days/week for 12 weeks
on a motor-driven treadmill with an 8^0 incline at a speed of 28
meters/minute for 60 minutes each day. These animals were young and
still growing. The final body weights are presented in Table III.
This relatively mild exercise program produced a 15% difference in
weights between the trained and sedentary groups.
The difference in body weights between the trained and sedentary
animals was almost exclusively due to a lower amount of body fat in
the trained group. The weights of individual tissues are presented
in Table III. The trained animals have virtually no difference in
muscle or organ weights but have approximately 40% less body fat.
Individual adipose tissues range from 34 to 49% less than in the
sedentary animals. Other studies have examined the changes in the
composition of the total body with respect to water, protein, fat
and ash and the results are similar to those found with tissue
analysis. These studies found decreases in both the relative and
absolute amounts of body fat, plus an increase in the percentage of
FFB in growing (55,58,59) or adult (60) animals. Thus the difference in weights between sedentary and trained animals was almost
entirely due to lower body fat in the endurance trained animals.

As stated above, moderate aerobic exercise has little effect on weights of other tissues (Table III). There are some reports of increased heart weights due to aerobic exercise (54,61); however, most studies found only changes in functional parameters such as heart rate and stroke volume (54,62). Skeletal muscles directly associated with performing aerobic exercise generally do not increase in size (63). Instead, changes in skeletal muscles occur at the cellular level through increases in mitochondrial number and size and increases in oxidative capacity (64). The increase in the weight of the adrenal gland is a consistent finding during aerobic training and reflects that exercise is a stress to the body which generates an endocrine response (54).

The study presented in Table III demonstrates that aerobic exercise alters energy balance and reduces body fat. The mechanism for this response was addressed by Mayer (65,66). He reported that exercise influenced energy balance by increasing caloric expenditure and by reducing appetite. Other studies have also reported that aerobic exercise produced appetite suppression, particularly in male rats (59,60). These investigators suggested that the effect was related to the intensity and duration of the exercise program. The food intake data for the study described in Table III are presented in Table IV and appear to support this conclusion. After only

Table IV. Average Daily Food Intake

Group	Weeks of Training	
	4	7
	(Kcal/day)	
Sedentary	70.3 + 3.7	72.0 + 2.5
Trained	59.5 + 2.5*	73.3 + 4.6

Values are Means + SEM, n = 7, * $p < 0.05$.
(Quig and Layman, unpublished.)

4 weeks of training, animals consumed 15% less energy each day. However, after 7 weeks of training, the food intake of the trained animals had returned to normal. This finding is similar to the report of Applegate et al. (67) using a lower intensity exercise with obese rats. Thus negative energy balance can be produced during exercise due to increased energy expenditure, or decreased caloric intake, or both.

In contrast to male rats, female rats subjected to endurance training maintain body weight comparable to sedentary age controls by increasing food intake (65). However, while females maintain total body weight, exercise still produces the same effects on body composition. Thus in evaluating animal studies, it is important to remember that, during moderate to heavy exercise training, male rats experience appetite suppression and lose body weight and body fat. While under similar conditions, female rats will maintain body

weight by increasing food intake. Female rats still experience the
decrease in both the absolute and relative amounts of body fat but
may have a small increase in LBM.

Body Composition Changes Due to Diet and Exercise

Lay publications are inundated with fad diets designed to reduce
body weight "quickly and easily" using a variety of caloric
restrictions (68). Most individuals attempt to produce a negative
energy balance and reduce body weight by decreasing food intake.
The advantage of using food restriction is that it accelerates the
rate of weight loss. However, the enthusiasm for these diets
dissipates after two or three weeks and the weight is regained. In
addition, it is unclear if the weight loss generated by these diets
produces any improvement in body composition.

There are numerous studies involving humans or animals that
have examined the effects of caloric restriction on the composition
of weight loss (69,70,71,72). These studies indicate that food
restriction causes decreases in body weight and body fat, and that
the magnitude of these losses is proportional to the length and the
severity of the food deprivation. There are also substantial losses
of skeletal muscle and organ tissues (71,72). Assuming the goal is
to optimize health, then the objective is to decrease body fat
content, and maintain FFB weight which will maximize the benefits of
weight loss. Therefore, it is important to examine the specific
effects of dieting on body composition.

During the early phase of dieting, water accounts for a large
percentage of the weight lost (69). Hence, the rate of weight loss
is much higher during the first few days of diet modification,
because the caloric density of the weight loss is low. After the
initial adaptation to a lower caloric intake, the weight loss is
derived predominantly from stores of body fat plus losses of FFB to
provide sufficient amino acids for essential protein synthesis and
gluconeogenesis (73). These losses occur at a relatively constant
ratio with FFB estimated to contribute 35-50% of the weight loss
(14). This ratio differs depending on the percentage of body fat
and age of the animal, but the ratio remains approximately constant
for an animal throughout a period of food restriction (72). Thus
weight loss by diet alone will decrease body weight, but produces
little improvement in body composition.

Weight loss produced by dietary restriction in combination with
aerobic exercise appears to provide a more optimal weight loss based
on improvements in body composition. The amount of body fat lost is
proportional to the caloric deficit (i.e., the decrease in intake
plus the increase in expenditure), but the composition of the weight
loss is also dependent on the amount of FFB lost. The loss of FFB
is reduced by exercise which selectively maintains muscle mass.
Thus, weight loss associated with exercise becomes more specifically
loss of body fat (60).

These data suggest that the optimal regimen for reducing body
fat is a combination of diet restriction and aerobic exercise. The
components of an exercise program are defined by the parameters
intensity, duration, and frequency. Intensity refers to the vigor
of the activity and can be defined by heart rate. Duration
describes the length of the workout, and frequency indicates the

number of sessions each week. The primary objective of an exercise program designed to improve body composition is to maximize the amount of energy expended and to do so under conditions that will optimize mobilization and utilization of fat as the energy source. To most effectively accomplish these objectives, it is imperative that the exercise intensity be moderate. A moderate exercise program consists of maintaining an exercise heart rate of 130-150 beats per minute (b/min) in the 20- to 50-year age range (110-130 b/min in the 50- to 80-year range) for 30 to 45 minutes per session with a frequency of 3 to 4 days per week (74). This program will utilize approximately 1000 Kcal per week and lead to fat loss. The type of exercise should require use of a major portion of the muscle mass. Walking, jogging, bicycling, and swimming are normally activities of choice. In the severely obese, bicycling and swimming are particularly useful activities since they are non-weight bearing and thus produce less orthopedic stress.

Summary

Obesity is a major health problem in the United States. It is estimated that the body composition of one in every three Americans contains an excessive amount of body fat which may predispose these individuals to increased risk of high blood pressure, heart disease, diabetes, gout, and other adult diseases. Modification of body composition, and specifically reduction of body fat, requires a decrease in food intake and/or an increase in exercise. These changes in the balance of energy intake and expenditure will reduce body weight. The actual composition of the weight loss is dependent on the level of dietary restriction and the amount of physical activity. Weight loss due to "dieting" alone has a relatively small effect on body composition because body fat and muscle are lost in approximately equal amounts. Dieting plus aerobic exercise decreases body weight by increasing the use of energy stored in body fat, but also serves to maintain the muscle mass through increased usage.

A prescription for modification of body composition must consider the intensity, duration, and frequency of exercise as well as the nutritional intake. The general guidelines for such a prescription include reduction of dietary intake by 500-1000 Calories each day with a minimum of three sessions of aerobic exercise each week. This program should produce a slow weight loss of approximately one pound per week and should maintain the daily food intake above 1200 Calories, which is considered the minimum for a nutritionally adequate diet.

The exercise program should entail three or four sessions of aerobic exercise per week with each session lasting 30-40 minutes. The desired intensity of these activities can be best gauged by heart rate, which should be in a range of 130-150 beats per minute. This program is designed to reduce body fat and maintain muscle mass. Use of the exercise alone will serve to maintain body composition and prevent the age-related increases in body fat frequently observed in adults.

Literature Cited

1. Hannon, B. M. & Lohman, T. G. (1978) The energy cost of overweight in the United States. Amer. J. Pub. Health 68, 765-767.

2. Buskirk, E. R. (1971) Obesity. In: Physiological Basis of Rehabilitation Medicine (Downey, J. A. & Darling, R. C., eds.), pp. 229-242, W. B. Saunders, Philadelphia.

3. McArdle, W. D., Katch, F. I. & Katch, V. L. (1981) Exercise Physiology: Energy, Nutrition, and Performance. Lea & Febiger, Philadelphia, pp. 405-424.

4. Coates, T., Killen, J. & Slinkard, L. (1982) Parent participation in a treatment program for overweight adolescents. Inter. J. Eating Disorders 1, 37-48.

5. Ylitalo, V. (1981) Treatment of obese school children. Acta Paediat. Scand. (Suppl. 290), 1-108.

6. AAHPERD Health Related Physical Fitness Test Manual. (1980) AAHPERD Publication, Reston, VA.

7. Pate, R. R., Ross, J. G., Dotson, C. O. & Gilbert, G. G. (1985) The natural children and youth fitness study. The new norms: a comparison with the 1980 AAHPERD norms. J. Phy. Educ., Rec. & Dance 56, 70-72.

8. Johnson, F. E., Hamill, D. V. & Lemeshow, S. (1972) Skinfold thickness of children 6-11 years (Series II, No. 120). U.S. Center for Health Statistics, Washington.

9. Johnson, F. E., Hamill, D. V. & Lemeshow, S. (1974) Skinfold thickness of youth 12-17 years (Series II, No. 132). U.S. Center for Health Statistics, Washington.

10. Kolata, G. (1985) Obesity declared a disease. Science 227, 1019-1020.

11. Warner, W. A. & Garrett, L. P. (1968) The obese patient and anesthesia. J. Am. Med. Assoc. 205, 102-103.

12. Wilson, R.H.L. & Wilson, N. L. (1969) Obesity and respiratory stress. J. Am. Diet. Assoc. 55, 465-469.

13. Lowrey, G. H. (1978) Growth and Development of Children, 7th ed., Yearbook Medical Publishers, Inc., Chicago, pp. 409-444.

14. Brownell, K. D. & Wadden, T. A. (1983) Behavioral and self-help treatments. In: Obesity (Greenwood, M.R.C., ed.), pp. 39-64, Churchill Livingstone, New York.

15. Fellingham, G. W., Roundy, E. S., Fisher, A. G. & Bryce, G. R. (1978) Caloric cost of walking and running. Med. Sci. Sports 10, 132-136.

16. Leon, A. S., Conrad, J., Hunninghake, D. B. & Serfass, R. (1979) Effects of a vigorous walking program on body composition and carbohydrate and lipid metabolism of obese young men. Am. J. Clin. Nutr. 32, 1776-1787.

17. Boileau, R. A. & Lohman, T. G. (1977) The measurement of human physique and its effect on physical performance. Orthoped. Clin. N. Amer. 8, 563-581.

18. Wilmore, J. (1983) Body composition in sport and exercise: directions for future research. Med. Sci. Sports Exerc. 15, 21-31.

19. Grande, F. (1968) Energy balance and body composition changes: a critical study of three recent publications. Ann. Int. Med. 68, 467-480.

20. Moody, D. L., Kollias, J. & Buskirk, E. R. (1969) The effect of a moderate exercise program on body weight and skinfold thickness in overweight college women. Med. Sci. Sports 1, 74-80.

21. Wilmore, J. H., Royce, J., Girandola, R. N., Katch, F. I. & Katch, V. L. (1970) Body composition changes with a 10-week program of jogging. Med. Sci. Sports 2, 113-117.

22. Boileau, R. A., Buskirk, E. R., Horstman, D. H., Mendez, J. & Nicholas, W. C. (1971) Body composition changes in obese and lean men during physical conditioning. Med. Sci. Sports 3, 183-189.

23. Björntorp, P. (1983) Physiological and clinical aspect of exercise in obese persons. In: Exercise and Sport Sciences Reviews (Terjung, R. L., ed.), pp. 159-180, Franklin Institute Press, Philadelphia.

24. Oscai, L. B. (1984) Recent progress in understanding obesity. In: Exercise and Health, American Academy of Physical Education Paper No. 17 (Eckert, H. M. & Montoye, H. J., eds.), pp. 42-48, Human Kinetics Publishers, Champaign, IL.

25. Oscai, L. B. (1973) The role of exercise in weight control. In: Exercise and Sport Sciences Reviews, vol. 1 (Wilmore, J. H., ed.), pp. 103-125, Academic Press, New York.

26. Behnke, A. R. & Wilmore, J. H. (1974) Evaluation and Regulation of Body Build and Composition, Prentice-Hall, Inc., Englewood Cliffs, NJ.

27. Boileau, R. A., Lohman, T. G. & Slaughter, M. H. Exercise and body composition in children and youth. Scand. J. Sports Sci., in press.

28. Keys, A., Brozek, J., Henschel, A., Mickelsen, O. & Taylor,
    H. L. (1950) The Biology of Human Starvation, Vols. I & II.
    University of Minnesota Press, Minneapolis.

29. Zuti, W. B. & Golding, L. A. (1976) Comparing diet and
    exercise as weight reduction tools. Physic. Sports Med. 4,
    49-53.

30. Brozek, J., Grande, F., Anderson, J. T. & Keys, A. (1963)
    Densitometric analysis of body composition: revision of some
    quantitative assumptions. Ann. N.Y. Acad. Sci. 110, 113-140.

31. Forbes, G. B. & Hursh, J. B. (1963) Age and sex trends in
    lean body mass calculated from K-40 measurements with a note on
    the theoretical basis for the procedure. Ann. N.Y. Acad. Sci.
    110, 255-263.

32. Keys, A. & Brozek, J. (1953) Body fat in adult man. Physiol.
    Rev. 33, 245-325.

33. Lohman, T. G., Boileau, R. A. & Slaughter, M. H. (1984) Body
    composition in children and youth. In: Advances in Pediatric
    Sports Sciences (Boileau, R. A., ed.), vol. 1, pp. 29-57, Human
    Kinetics Publishers, Champaign, IL.

34. Cohn, S. H., Ellis, K. J. & Wallach, S. (1974) In vivo
    neutron activation analysis: clinical potential in body
    composition studies. Am. J. Med. 57, 683-686.

35. Nyboer, J. (1972) Workable volume and flow concepts of
    bio-segments by electrical impedance plethysmography T.-T.-T.
    J. Life Sci. 2, 1-13.

36. Presta, E., Wang, J., Harrison, G. G., Björntorp, P., Harker,
    W. H. & Van Itallie, T. B. (1983) Measurement of total body
    electrical conductivity: a new method for estimation of body
    composition. Am. J. Clin. Nutr. 37, 735-739.

37. Lohman, T. G. (1984) Research progress in validation of
    laboratory methods of assessing body composition. Med. Sci.
    Sports Exerc. 16, 596-603.

38. Anderson, E. C. (1963) Three-component body composition
    analysis based on potassium and water determinations. Ann.
    N.Y. Acad. Sci. 110, 189-210.

39. Behnke, A. R., Feen, B. G. & Welham, W. C. (1942) Specific
    gravity of healthy men. J. Am. Med. Assoc. 118, 495-498.

40. Buskirk, E. R. (1961) Underwater weighing and body density:
    a review of procedures. In: Techniques for Measuring Body
    Composition (Brozek, J. & Henschel, A., eds.), pp. 90-106,
    National Academy of Sciences and National Research Council,
    Washington, DC.

41. Morales, M. F., Rathbun, E. N., Smith, R. E. & Pace, N. (1945) Studies on body composition II. Theoretical considerations regarding the major body tissue components, with suggestions for application to man. J. Biol. Chem. 158, 677–684.

42. Siri, W. E. (1961) Body composition from fluid spaces and density: analysis of methods. In: Techniques for Measuring Body Composition (Brozek, J. & Henschel, A., eds.), pp. 223–244, National Academy of Sciences and National Research Council, Washington, DC.

43. Parizkova, J. (1961) Total body fat and skinfold thickness in children. Metab. 10, 794–809.

44. Boileau, R. A., Wilmore, J. H., Lohman, T. G., Slaughter, M. H. & Riner, W. F. (1981) Estimation of body density from skinfold thicknesses, body circumferences and skeletal widths in boys aged 8 to 11 years: comparison of two samples. Human Biol. 53, 575–592.

45. Heald, F. P., Hunt, E. E., Schwartz, R., Cook, C. D., Elliot, D. & Vajda, B. (1963) Measures of body fat and hydration in adolescent boys. Pediat. 31, 226–239.

46. Young, C. M., Bogan, A. D., Roe, D. A. & Lutwak, L. (1968) Body composition of preadolescent and adolescent girls IV. Body water and creatinine. J. Am. Diet. Assoc. 53, 579–587.

47. Boileau, R. A., Lohman, T. G., Slaughter, M. H., Ball, T. E., Going, S. B. & Hendrix, M. K. (1984) Hydration of the fat-free body in children during maturation. Human Biol. 56, 651–666.

48. Lohman, T. G., Slaughter, M. H., Boileau, R. A., Bunt, J. & Lussier, L. (1984) Bone mineral measurements and their relation to body density in children, youth and adults. Human Biol. 56, 667–679.

49. Fomon, S. J., Haschke, F., Ziegler, E. E. & Nelson, S. E. (1982) Body composition of reference children from birth to age 10 years. Am. J. Clin. Nutr. 35, 1169–1175.

50. Boileau, R. A., Lohman, T. G., Slaughter, M. H. & Bunt, J. C. (1984) Variability in the fat-free body composition of children. Fed. Proc. 43, 861.

51. Norris, A. H., Lundy, T. & Shock, N. W. (1963) Trends in selected indices of body composition in men between the ages of 30 and 80 years. Ann. N.Y. Acad. Sci. 110, 623–639.

52. Mazess, R. B. (1982) On aging bone loss. Clin. Orthoped. 165, 239–252.

53. Slaughter, M. H., Lohman, T. G., Boileau, R. A., Stillman, R. J., Van Loan, M., Horswill, C. A. & Wilmore, J. H. (1984) Influence of maturation on relationship of skinfolds to body density: a cross-sectional study. Human Biol. 56, 681-689.

54. Tipton, C. M., Terjung, R. L. & Barnard, R. J. (1968) Response of thyroidectomized rats to training. Am. J. Physiol. 215, 1137-1142.

55. Crews, E. L., Fuge, K. W., Oscai, L. B., Holloszy, J. O. & Shank, R. E. (1969) Weight, food intake, and body composition: effects of exercise and protein deficiency. Am. J. Physiol. 216, 359-363.

56. Faulkner, J. A., Maxwell, L. C., Brook, G. A. & Lieberman, D. A. (1971) Adaptation of guinea pig plantaris muscle fibers to endurance training. Am. J. Physiol. 221, 291-297.

57. Dudley, G. A., Abraham, W. M. & Terjung, R. L. (1982) Influence of exercise intensity and duration on biochemical adaptations in skeletal muscle. J. Appl. Physiol. 53, 844-850.

58. Pitts, G. C. (1956) Body fat accumulation in the guinea pig. Am. J. Physiol. 185, 41-48.

59. Jones, E. M., Montoye, H. J, Johnson, P. B., Martin, S.M.J.M., Van Huss, W. D. & Cederquist, D. C. (1964) Effects of exercise and food restriction on serum cholesterol and liver lipids. Am. J. Physiol. 207, 460-466.

60. Oscai, L. B. & Holloszy, J. O. (1969) Effects of weight changes produced by exercise, food restriction, or overeating on body composition. J. Clin. Invest. 48, 2124-2128.

61. Oscai, L. B., Mole, P. A., Krusack, L. M. & Holloszy, J. O. (1973) Detailed body composition analysis on female rats subjected to a program of swimming. J. Nutr. 103, 412-418.

62. Harpur, R. P. (1980) The rat as a model for physical fitness studies. Comp. Biochem. Physiol. 66A, 553-574.

63. Terjung, R. L. (1976) Muscle fiber involvement during training of different intensities and durations. Am. J. Physiol. 230, 946-950.

64. Holloszy, J. O. & Booth, F. W. (1976) Biochemical adaptations to endurance exercise in muscle. Ann. Rev. Physiol. 38, 273-291.

65. Mayer, J., Marshall, N. B., Vitale, J. J., Christensen, J. H., Mashayekhi, M. B. & Stare, F. J. (1954) Exercise, food intake and body weight in normal rats and genetically obese adult mice. Am. J. Physiol. 177, 544-548.

66. Mayer, J., Roy, P. & Mitra, K. P. (1956) Relation between caloric intake, body weight, and physical work. Am. J. Clin. Nutr. 4, 169-175.

67. Applegate, E. A., Upton, D. E. & Stern, J. S. (1984) Exercise and detraining: effect on food intake, adiposity and lipogenesis in Osborne-Mendel rats made obese by a high fat diet. J. Nutr. 114, 447-459.

68. Stern, J. S. (1983) Diet and exercise. In: Obesity (Greenwood, M.R.C., ed.), pp. 65-84, Churchill Livingstone, New York.

69. Keys, A., Brozek, J., Henschel, A., Mickelsen, O. & Taylor, H. L. (1950) The Biology of Human Starvation, vols. I & II, University of Minnesota Press, Minneapolis.

70. Young, V. R. (1971) The physiology of starvation. Sci. Amer. 225, 14-21.

71. Goodman, M. N., Lowell, B., Belur, E. & Ruderman, N. B. (1984) Sites of protein conservation and loss during starvation: influence of adiposity. Am. J. Physiol. 246, E383-E390.

72. Glore, S. R., Layman, D. K. & Bechtel, P. J. (1984) Skeletal muscle and fat pad losses in male and female Zucker lean and obese rats after prolonged starvation. Nutr. Rep. Int. 29, 797-805.

73. Cahill, G. F. (1970) Starvation in man. New Eng. J. Med., pp. 668-675.

74. Pollock, M. L. (1973) The quantification of endurance training programs. In Exercise and Sport Sciences Reviews, Vol. 1 (Wilmore, J. H., ed.), pp. 155-188, Academic Press, New York.

RECEIVED June 12, 1985

Glossary

Anthropometry: study of comparative measurements of the body, including height or length, circumferences, and skinfolds.

Apoliproteins: the surface proteins of lipoproteins; apoliproteins AI and AII are the major apoliproteins of HDL; apo CII is a lipoprotein present on chylomicrons and VLDL which activates the enzyme lipoprotein lipase.

Black-Globe temperature: the temperature inside a hollow copper sphere 15.2 cm (6 in.) in diameter painted matt-black on the outside and containing a thermometer inserted so that its sensing unit is at the center of the sphere. This temperature is a measure of the intensity of radiant heat from the surroundings or the sun.

Calories: a unit of heat; the quantity of energy required to raise the temperature of 1 Kg of water 1 C. Calorie with a capital "C" is equivalent to kilocalorie (Kcal) and is used in nutrition to describe energy intake and expenditure.

Chylomicron: triglyceride rich lipoprotein that transports lipids of dietary origin to peripheral tissues.

Coronary Heart Disease (CHD): atherosclerosis; a particular type of hardening of the arteries involving infiltration of fatty materials into the arterial wall.

Dehydration: the process of depletion of body water from deprivation or loss.

Dipsogen: a substance that stimulates thirst.

Dry-bulb temperature: the temperature indicated by a dry-bulb thermometer, shielded from the sun, with a diameter large enough to allow free passage of air around the bulb; the actual temperature of the air.

Double-blind experiment: experimental design where the subjects do not know whether they are receving the experimental treatment or a placebo.

Fat free body: the remainder of the body excluding all lipids or fats.

Glycogenolysis: the breakdown of glycogen to glucose.

Gluconeogenesis: synthesis of glucose from non-carbohydrate precursors such as amino acids.

High density lipoprotein (HDL): an antiatherogenic lipoprotein that facilitates the removal of cholesterol from tissues for subsequent catabolism.

Hypernatremia: increase in the plasma sodium concentration above the normal level.

Hyperosmotemia: increase in the plasma osmolar (salt) concentration above normal level.

Hyperproteinemia: increase in the plasma (total) protein concentration above normal level.

Hypervolemia: increase in the plasma volume above the normal level.

Hypohydration: an equilibrium level of total body water below the normal volume.

Hypovolemia: reduction in the plasma volume below the normal level.

In vitro: in the test tube; usually refers to chemical reactions occurring in a test tube.

In vivo: in the living being; usually refers to chemical processes occuring within the body.

Ischemic Heart disease: inadequate circulation of blood to the heart muscle.

Lean body mass (LBM): the mass of the body excluding the adipose tissues; LBM is the same as FFB plus approximately 3% essential fat contained in cell membranes.

Low density Lipoprotein (LPL): a lipoprotein that transports cholesterol to tissues; associated with increased risk of coronary heart disease.

Myocardial infarction (MI): heart attack; death of the heart muscle due to a blood clot in a coronary artery.

Splanchnic: viseral; organs of the digestive, circulatory, respiratory, and endocrine systems.

Turnover: the continuous processes of synthesis and breakdown; often used to describe the steady-state of protein.

Very low density lipoprotein (VLDL): a triglyceride rich lipoprotein that transports lipid to tissues and serves as a precursor of LDL.

VO_2 max: maximum oxygen consumption.

Wet–bulb globe temperature index: a mathematical expression
    comprised of the dry–bulb, wet bulb, and black–globe tem–
    peratures, which indicates the combined effects of tem–
    perature, humidity, air movement, and thermal radiation
    as an environmental stress.

Wet–bulb temperature: the temperature indicated by a wet–bulb
    thermometer where the bulb is covered by a thin cotton
    or muslin sleeve, wetted with distilled water, and air
    is drawn over the bulb in a velocity of at least 107 meters/
    minute (350 feet/min).

Author Index

Subject Index

Production and indexing by Keith B. Belton
Jacket design by Pamela Lewis

Elements typeset by Hot Type Ltd., Washington, D.C.
Printed and bound by Maple Press Co., York, Pa.